BODY
LIBERATION

BODY LIBERATION

Freeing Your Body
for Greater
Self-Acceptance,
Health, and
Sexual Satisfaction

Emily Coleman
Betty Edwards

Published by
J.P. Tarcher, Inc., Los Angeles

Distributed by St. Martin's Press, Inc., New York

Copyright © 1977 By Emily Coleman and Betty Edwards
All rights reserved
Library of Congress Catalog Card Number: 75-32854
Publisher's ISBN: 0-87477-059-9
Distributor's ISBN: 312-90438-X
Manufactured in the United States of America
Published by J. P. Tarcher, Inc.
9110 Sunset Blvd., Los Angeles, CA 90069
Published simultaneously in Canada by Macmillan of Canada
70 Bond St., Toronto, Canada M5B IX3

Dedicated to

My partners, Betty Edwards in writing and
Keith Tombrink in the Man-Woman Institute;
they comfort me when I think I know nothing
and challenge me when I think I know everything.
—*Emily Coleman*

Ruth, my mother, who left me a dream,
and Susie, my stepmother, who helped me fulfill it.
—*Betty Edwards*

Acknowledgments

We appreciate all the help and encouragement we received from those at the J. P. Tarcher Company who were associated with us during the writing of this book.

We are particularly grateful for the close working relationship we had with our publisher, Jeremy Tarcher. Through countless hours of discussion he helped us find our direction.

We are indebted to the many authorities in many fields who granted us personal interviews. While space limitations prevent us from listing them individually, their contributions to the book have been invaluable. We want to give a very special *Thank you* to the following people who helped us in some very special ways.

Dr. William Hartman and Mrs. Marilyn Fithian, director and co-director of the Center for Marital and Sexual Studies in Long Beach, California, who generously shared the facilities of their clinic, their time, and their knowledge with us.

Ed Lange, who made the facilities of Elysium available to us and our friends for research, who aided us with valuable suggestions, and whose pioneering work in the field of body liberation helped make our book possible.

Bill Hardwick, owner of Mountain Terrace Ranch, and Dick and Thelma Manning of Olive Dell Nudist Resort, who allowed us to visit their facilities and interview their guests.

The participants in Emily's Brave Nude World workshop in Santa Barbara in the summer of 1975 who allowed us to tape a session and put their private thoughts and feelings about their bodies on paper (under different names, of course).

Kathi Wundes and Jeanette Watson, who patiently typed and retyped our sometimes hard to read manuscript, and Judy Ford and Joanne Schneider at Tam's stationers who copied and copied and copied.

And most especially our friends who aided us in some or all of the following ways—by discussing ideas with us, by participating in some of our activities, and by giving us moral support and encouragement when we needed it—Kathleen Varley, Irv Howard, Glenn Putnam, John Kern, Roy and Betsy Covert, Stanton and Carol Booth, Frank and Betty McGill, Dick Nazro, Ed Ohm, June Forrester, Richard and Doris Littrell, Bob Miller, Hal Winters, Joanne Norris, Wright Jackson, Violet Oaklander, Bill Mueller, and Keith Tombrink.

Contents

1   The Promise of Body Liberation   1

PART ONE
TOWARD BODY PRIDE

2   The Victorian Inheritance   14
3   Taking Charge of Your Body and Yourself   24
4   Integrating Your Mind and Body   42
5   Breaking the Seeing and Touching Taboo   58
6   Being Born Again   69
7   Realizing Body Joy   78
8   Going Bare with Children   90
9   Going Bare with Your Sexual Partner   103

PART TWO
BEYOND BODY TABOOS

10   Going Bare with Others   122
11   Accepting Yourself in a Brave Nude World   135
12   Nude Beaches, Resorts, and Travel Tours   147
13   Growth Centers: Esalen, Elysium, and Sandstone   158
14   Body Joy with Others   172
15   The Politics of Going Bare   197

Epilogue: Declaration of Body Independence   205
Appendix: Where to Go for More Information   213
Bibliography   219
Index   226

Chapter 1
The Promise of Body Liberation

> Legs!
> How we have suffered each other,
> never meeting the standards of magazines
>   or official measurements.
>
>   Kathleen Fraser,
>   *Poem in Which My Legs Are Accepted*

Most of us dislike at least one part of our bodies. If it isn't chunky legs, it's a fat stomach or narrow shoulders or bags under the eyes. The possibilities are endless. Most of us, in fact, dislike many parts of our bodies and like very few parts. If asked to list positive things about our bodies, few of us can think of as many as half a dozen and many are hard pressed to come up with anything at all. However, if asked to list our dislikes, most of us could fill a page, many could fill several pages, and some could write a book. How about you? Consider the following list and check off the statements that you agree with.

Body Dislikes

I am too short.
I am too tall.
I am too fat.
I am too skinny.
My posture is bad.
I have too much hair on my body.
I have too little hair on my body.

The hair on my head is too thin (or the wrong color).
I am bald.
My skin is oily (or dry, or pimply, or splotchy, or rough, or the pores are too large).
My eyes are too close together (or too far apart).
I have bags under my eyes.
My teeth are crooked (or have gaps or are yellowed).
My ears stick out (or are misshapen).
My nose is too big (or too long or too flat).
My lips are too thin (or too thick or not well-shaped).
My mouth is too big.
I have a double chin.
My neck is too long (or too short or wrinkled).
My shoulders are too narrow (or too wide or lopsided).
My arms aren't muscular enough (or are too muscular).
My upper arms are flabby.
My hands are rough.
My fingers are short and fat.
My chest caves in.
My breasts are too big (or too small, or sag, or are too far apart or too close together, or the nipples are too large or too small).
I have a thick waist.
My stomach is too fat.
My hip bones stick out.
My hips are too wide.
My thighs are too fat (or too skinny).
My bottom is too broad (or too fat).
My penis is too small.
My testicles hang down too low.
My legs are too short (or too long or too large or too skinny).
My knees are knobby.
I have varicose veins.
My feet are too big.

Add anything else you dislike about your appearance. Now list what you do like and compare the two lists.

Was your list of body-dislikes longer than your list of body-likes? If so, you have lots of company. According to a 1973 *Psychology Today* survey of 62,000 readers (a highly educated and sophisticated readership), only 45 percent of the women and 55 percent of the men had a positive body image; that is, they were completely satisfied with their appearance.

Most of us are unhappy not only with the way we look but also with the way our bodies behave. They don't always do what we want them to do. Time after time, they fail us by developing itches, aches, and pains; by giving off odors or secretions or perspiration; by producing unwanted changes in skin and hair and scalp. Energy falters; muscles behave awkwardly; tics and nervous mannerisms arise; we develop gas; and either we can't wake up in the morning or fall asleep at night. When our bodies won't work so long or so hard as we would like them to, they make us feel guilty or uncomfortable, accusing us of wasting time daydreaming or staring out the window.

Sometimes we don't even notice how much our bodies annoy us. We are not consciously aware of our assumption that our bodies are unattractive, a nuisance, and impossible to control. We take precautions against certain physical ills, but leave our bodies unexamined because we are prejudiced against them. At worst, like some of our most feared diseases, body prejudice can do great harm. At best, like some less dangerous maladies, body prejudice limits our joy, our freedom, and our productivity—every day.

THE HIGH COST OF BODY PREJUDICE

As individuals and as a culture we demonstrate our body prejudice in the following ways:

    1. We pick such ideal standards for good looks that the majority of bodies can seldom, if ever, measure up.

    2. We fail to seek knowledge of body functions—in fact, they embarrass us.

    3. We suppress strong emotions and thereby restrict our ability to express any emotion.

    4. We fail to allow ourselves many simple sensory delights, believing it is somehow not quite right to experience pleasure through our bodies.

How can we say people are prejudiced against their bodies, you might ask, when so much attention and so much money are spent on them? Probably the greatest percentage of the average person's income is spent on products for the body—clothing, food, cosmetics, exercise equipment or activities, medical treatment, prescriptions, and over-the-counter drugs. But most of this money is not spent with the attitude that a body is a friend we understand, trust, care about, and want to make happy. Instead, money is spent with the idea that the body is an adversary, an unreliable object that is given pleasure only as bribery or appeasement. A body is something to be prodded, pushed, pummeled, deprived, forced, and treated with chemicals in the attempt to get it to shape up, to conform to prevailing (and unrealistic) standards of beauty and performance. When the body doesn't shape up, we disguise or conceal it.

How does discontent with the way we see our bodies affect our lives? When most of us look in the mirror we do not see ourselves as others see us. Just as we notice the weeds in our own backyard and the flowers in our neighbor's, the negative aspects of our bodies loom in the foreground and are magnified. On the other hand, we overlook or minimize our positive features. This unrealistic body image is harmful.

Body image—the way we visualize our bodies, what we see in the mirror, and the way we feel about what we see—is an important part of self-esteem. Psychologists have shown time and again the correlation between negative body image and low self-esteem, and between positive body image and high self-esteem. Surveys have shown that men and women who have above-average body images (but not necessarily objectively better bodies) also have above-average self-esteem and consider themselves more assertive, likable, and intelligent than the average person.

The attitude with which we face life each day depends on how much we value ourselves, and the way we see our body is the way we see ourselves. As a result of a negative body image we go through life as if we weren't worthwhile. We may spend a lot of money trying to improve our appearance in the hope of liking ourselves better. But the money isn't going to do a bit of good if our dislike of what we see is based on a lack of self-acceptance. When we see ourselves as less than we are we fail to discover, develop, or utilize our abilities. Thus, both as individuals and as a culture the cost to us of lack of body acceptance becomes staggering.

When we are unable to see the beauty in our own bodies—just as they are—we cannot see the beauty in other bodies, in other people—just as they are. We frequently fail to start new relationships because we do not consider ourselves worthwhile. We may destroy existing relationships because, not liking ourselves, we cannot like others. Unrealistic body standards and body prejudices affect our relationships in other ways, too. To the extent that we undervalue the average human body, we will overvalue the comparatively rare number of people who meet our cultural standards of beauty; we will attribute them with unreal and possibly undeserved qualities. Here are a number of ways we overvalue physical beauty in this society.

Highly attractive men and women are assumed to be superior in character, as well as in looks. One study showed students photographs of other students divided into categories of high, medium, and low attractiveness. The highly attractive males and females in the photos were seen as "more curious, complex, perceptive, confident, assertive, happy, active, amiable, candid, serious, pleasure-seeking, outspoken, and flexible" than the less attractive men and women. In another study using the same photographs, highly attractive males and females were seen as having more inner control over their own behavior and as being less influenced by others.

Beautiful women are "put on a pedestal" in our society. Dr. Merrill E. Sarty, from the University of Southern California School of Medicine, asked people ranging in age from 17 to 60 to rate attractive and less attractive women on their looks and then speculate on what their personalities and sexual attitudes were like. From more than 2,000 responses, Sarty concluded that people believe beautiful women have sex more often and enjoy it more, tend to marry later and have smaller families, and are more intelligent and liberated than their less beautiful sisters.

Adults make judgments about attractive children that can influence the way they treat the children. Psychologists Ellen Berscheid and Elaine Walster asked 400 fifth-grade teachers to examine records (of attendance, grades, work habits, etc.) and photographs of students and evaluate them in a number of ways. Although their records were similar, some of the students were physically attractive, others unattractive. Both male and female teachers believed the attractive students had higher IQs, better social relationships, higher educational potential, and more concerned and involved parents. The effect of evaluating physically attractive young children in this way may often be that these children receive special attention from their teachers. As a result this special attention may confirm the teachers' predictions of greater accomplishments from these students.

Our cultural bias in favor of good looks is so strong that just being with a good-looking person automatically confers status upon the person accompanying him or her. Experimenters introduced men (of comparable appearance), accompanied by dates, to other people, who then evaluated the men. The men with attractive women were rated more likable and of better character than the men with unattractive women. And the men themselves expected this positive evaluation if they had an attractive partner.

Studies from three different universities show that *college students, in making judgments about the opposite sex, rely heavily on their first impressions.* Students were matched with blind dates at a dance and were later asked to evaluate their dates in a variety of ways. Both men and women tended to use physical attractiveness as the main basis for evaluating their dates and for deciding if they wanted to go out with them again.

Studies like these show that we not only make snap judgments about people on the basis of their appearance but we also act upon these judgments. Many times, largely on the basis of people's looks, we decide whether or not to hire them, sit next to them on the bus, ask them to dance, acquit them of a crime, vote for them, give them a good grade, or simply get acquainted with them. While some of these decisions are inconsequential, others affect our lives in important ways (as in the selection of a mate, a friend, or an employee), and some can have national consequences (as in voting for a political candidate). In addition, we sometimes back away from people whose appearance puts us off, though these people could enrich our lives with their good qualities if we merely gave ourselves the time to discover what they were like.

While you may believe that you would be happier and that friends would come flocking to you if you were more beautiful, it just isn't so. Attractive people are often no happier or better adjusted than less attractive people. In fact, beautiful people tend to be just as discontented with their appearance as ordinary people—perhaps even more so.

In her body education workshops Emily Coleman has noted that the way people feel about their appearance usually has very little to do with the way they appear to others. This is particularly true of women, because our culture teaches women to believe they must be beautiful in order to be worthwhile and feminine. The self-worth of many beautiful women is tied up in their appearance and they feel they are never beautiful enough. Any physical flaw, no matter how minute (a mole, a frown line, an enlarged pore, an extra inch around the waist), can make a beautiful woman feel totally inadequate.

Nor do attractive men and women necessarily have better relationships with others. Women often suspect (sometimes with good reason) that men want to use them as status symbols. Beautiful women sometimes find relationships with other women difficult because of envy. Handsome men may not be taken seriously—people may assume they are lazy, narcissistic, Don Juans, or homosexuals. Women may even avoid handsome men because of these assumptions. In fact, attractive men and women are sometimes lonely because less attractive people of the opposite sex are afraid to approach them, believing them to be too busy, too popular, or too conceited to want anything to do with such an "ordinary" partner.

Attractive, unattractive, or just average, we are all deeply affected by our cultural attitudes toward physical beauty. Although our culture is not unique in having arbitrary standards of beauty (every society does), we are unique in the degree to which the mass media are constantly bombarding us with the ideals of physical perfection. Anyone who turns on the television, goes to a movie, picks up a magazine, or drives along a highway lined with billboards faces a constant and often unfavorable comparison to those who embody our standards of beauty. After all, how many women are so tall and slender as a fashion model or so large-breasted as the models in the men's magazines? And how many men have the broad shoulders and narrow hips our culture considers the masculine ideal?

Living in a society that looks down on bodies *as they are* condemns many of us to a chronic dissatisfaction that is likely to increase as we age and deviate more and more from the cultural ideal. In a culture that worships physical perfection, every line and wrinkle, every graying hair fills us with foreboding.

We have good reason to fear growing older. Our society is not kind to its elderly. Psychologist Seymour Fisher notes in *Body Consciousness: You Are What You Feel*, "The person of advanced years is made to feel that his body is despicable and that he is unworthy. He becomes a projective target for many of the fears and concerns of others." Instead of facing up to the fact that aging is a natural and inevitable part of the life cycle, we tend to regard it as a physical aberration. This may be one of the reasons older people are isolated and segregated in our society, sent to retirement homes or convalescent hospitals. We don't want to look at them, for it reminds us of what we believe is in store for us. Yet the symptoms of aging we see in others are by no means inevitable. People age faster than they need to when they live in a culture that tells them their bodies are inferior. Equating old with ugly, they give up at the first signs of old age. They feel discouraged and they do less. Then they feel terrible, attribute it to age, and fade into the woodwork. Or else, trying desperately to escape what they see as a terrible fate, if they can afford it they spend fortunes on face-lifts, or they put on too much makeup and wear clothes that are too youthful.

Chances are, many of the things we have been discussing have a familiar ring. Practically everyone has had experiences that point up our cultural obsession with physical attractiveness. However, few may recognize the extent of the damage that body prejudice—whether self-imposed or imposed by others—inflicts upon them.

To begin the process of liberating your own body, start by examining some of your body likes and dislikes. This will help you discover what values these critical judgments represent, what assumptions you are making because of them, and

THE PROMISE OF BODY LIBERATION

how these assumptions influence your life. Fill in the questionnaire below to help you discover some of your own associations between physical appearance and the other qualities people possess.

Body Appearance Questionnaire

List three things you particularly like about another person's body: (1) _____ , (2) _____ , (3) _____ .

List three things you particularly dislike about another person's body: (1) _____ , (2) _____ , (3) _____ .

Fill in the first blank in each statement below with the likes and dislikes you listed above. Then complete the statement for each like or dislike, showing the personality traits or attributes you associate with it.

For example:

When I see a person who has/is a big nose , I think he/she is vulgar and crude .

When I see a person who has/is fat , I think he/she is self-indulgent .

When I see a person who has/is firm thighs , I think he/she is athletic and sexy .

When I see a person who has/is slim, tapering fingers , I think he/she is high-class and artistic .

Now it's your turn:

When I see a person who has/is _____ , I think he/she _____ .

When I see a person who has/is _____ , I think he/she _____ .

When I see a person who has/is _____ , I think he/she _____ .

When I see a person who has/is _____ , I think he/she _____ .

When I see a person who has/is _____ , I think he/she _____ .

After completing the statement for *each* of your particular likes and dislikes, answer the following questions:
1. Do you know a person who has any of these physical characteristics but does *not* have the personality traits or attributes you associate with them?
2. When you see a stranger who has any of these physical characteristics, how do you behave toward him/her?
3. Do you have any of these characteristics yourself?
4. How does your having or lacking them affect your feelings about yourself?

SUGGESTIONS FOR BODY-LIBERATING ACTION

Write at the top of several sheets of blank paper:

THIS IS WHAT I LIKE ABOUT YOUR BODY
AND YOUR OVERALL APPEARANCE

Give one of these sheets to each of several close friends (it is especially helpful to include your sexual partner, your grown children, your parents). Tell them you are reading a book on body liberation, that you want to improve your body image and you need their help. Ask them to write on the sheet their honest appraisal of the positive aspects of your body. (Don't ask for negatives. You are overly aware of those already and are trying to achieve a more realistic balance.) Tell them to take their time and that you will ask them for the sheet in a day or two. When you pick up the lists, read them while you are still with your friends or family and discuss your feelings about what they have written with them. Chances are that doing this exercise will form a closer bond between you.

When you are finished, offer to fill out a sheet for each of them, if they wish it, but do not force the issue if they seem unwilling.

THE BENEFITS OF BODY LIBERATION AND
THE PROMISES OF THIS BOOK

The purpose of this book is to help you begin the process of liberating your body from your own body prejudice—from an intolerance of the way an average, normal body looks, functions, experiences, expresses, and enjoys bodily pleasure. These are the promises of body liberation.

1. *Liberating your body will increase your self-acceptance.* Your body is you. It is through bodily senses—seeing, hearing, tasting, smelling, and touching—that you know what is going on in your world. It is with your body that you communicate what goes on in your mind, heart, and soul. It is with your body that you take action. You cannot feel like a worthwhile person or accept your total self if you believe your basic biological being is substandard. Since lack of self-esteem is probably the biggest factor standing in the way of most people's happiness, almost every body-liberating exercise, concept, or technique in this book promotes self-acceptance in one form or another. Paradoxically, learning to accept your body *as it is* and to like yourself *as you are* can make it easier for you to change, if you choose to, some things about yourself that can be changed.

2. *Liberating your body will help you develop better relationships with others.* When you learn to like your own body, you will learn to get along better with the members of your own sex and to stop the destructive comparisons of your body to theirs. You will also be less apt to cling to, or be frightened by, members of the opposite sex. As you learn to like your physical appearance, you will expand the range of people you see as attractive and friendly. Recognizing that physical beauty comes in many forms other than slender, young, and sexy, you can become more tolerant of—and thus form better relationships with—those who differ from you in age, sex, and physique.

3. *Liberating your body will help you achieve better health.* Good health is more than the absence of disease; it is an overall sense of physical well-being. As you become more aware of all that affects your body, you will assume more responsibility for it. You will take better care of yourself, preventing discomfort and illness. Most important, you will recognize, believe, and act on the belief that vibrant good health requires you to express your feelings, live your values, determine a purpose for your life, and select friends who understand and respect you.

4. *Liberating your body will enhance your sex life.* Though most people believe they accept sex, many don't

know what acceptance is. Our so-called sexual revolution will not be truly effective until we rid ourselves of the prejudice that makes us ashamed of many of our body's functions and keeps us from being at ease with our own and our partner's body. Many of the ideas suggested in this book will help couples achieve the kind of comfort that makes sex exciting, uninhibited, and pleasurable.

    5. *Liberating your body will help you experience joy.* The only time many adults come close to a sense of physical joy is during orgasm. Even then, orgasm is more a sense of relief experienced primarily in the genitals rather than the deep, meaningful all-over pleasure it can be. The kind of joy we are talking about is the product of the full awakening of all your senses and involves the ability to be playful, exuberant, and spontaneous. Life can be much more than dealing with everyday problems—we can take full advantage of our many opportunities for pleasure.

    These are the main (but by no means the only) benefits of body liberation. It is first an individual process, but it is also a rapidly growing and important social trend. Body liberation is a movement whose time has come.

PART ONE
TOWARD BODY PRIDE

Chapter 2
The Victorian Inheritance

> The twentieth century may have learned to shorten bathing suits and get the body out into the light of day; it may have lightened clothing to allow freer movement and fuller display of the beguiling contours underneath; and it may have campaigned for sexual liberation. But it still has not fully come to terms with the human body.
>
> Stephen Kern,
> *Anatomy and Destiny:*
> *A Cultural History of the Human Body*

We weren't born with a prejudice toward bodies any more than we were born with a prejudice toward people of other cultures or religions. We learned our body prejudice in the process of growing up as members of a body-disparaging society. To understand how we have come to feel the way we do, it is essential to take a quick look at where our attitudes have come from. Let's start with a brief history of body attitudes in the Western world, particularly those derived from our religious tradition and from the relatively recent Victorian era.

PREJUDICE TOWARD NORMAL BODY FUNCTIONS

"For if ye live after the flesh, ye shall die: but if ye through the Spirit do mortify the deeds of the body, ye shall live." (*Romans* 8:13). These words of St. Paul hardly make us feel good about our bodies. But such early ideas about the sinfulness of the body were basic tenets of the Catholic Church. They remained largely undisturbed throughout the Protestant Reformation, and their influence still persists. The writings of John Calvin and Martin Luther, prime movers in the break from the authority of the Catholic Church, expressed similar contempt, if not loathing, for the human body:

> *Calvin:* The whole man from head to foot is thus, as it were, drenched in a flood of wickedness so that no part has remained without sin and so everything which springs from him is counted as sin.
>
> *Luther:* Our weakness lies not in our works but in our nature; our person, nature and entire being are corrupted through Adam's fall.

Who wouldn't be prejudiced against a body considered an evil vessel in which one was condemned to spend a lifetime? No wonder the idea arose that human beings are divided into two parts, body and soul, constantly at war with one another. In fact, in Christianity the needs of the body came to be viewed as impediments to the soul's salvation. Western man was taught to be proud of the activities of the spirit and mind but ashamed of the activities of the body, particularly sexual and excretory functions. Even in our less religious age we view many functions and needs of the body as shameful and certainly less noble than the needs of the mind.

The result of such attitudes is that, for example, you may find it less embarrassing to buy liquor or tranquilizers (supposedly for your mind) than to buy sanitary napkins or contraceptives (for your body). You may find it easier to talk to people about your emotional problems than about your hemorrhoidectomy. In mixed company, most people still find it somewhat difficult to excuse themselves to go to the toilet—as if they were about to do something shameful. Our language is full of euphemisms for where this natural function takes place: the "powder room," "little girls' " or "little boys' room," "bathroom," and "restroom."

Yet when it comes to other activities we are preoccupied with our bodies. We may, for example, buy soaps, lotions, sprays, and perfumes for our bodies, while ignoring an untidy personal life of unpaid debts, unfulfilled commitments, and unexamined goals.

What's more, designating some parts of the body and their functions as "bad" creates a sort of cultural schizophrenia, according to Dr. Herbert Otto, the founder and director of the National Center for the Exploration of Human Potential, in La Jolla, California: "When people are taught their bodies are bad and that nakedness in itself is sinful, they are bound to feel that parts of their bodies don't belong to them. Therefore, they cannot feel like whole people."

BODY PREJUDICE TOWARD FEELINGS AND PLEASURE

In addition to the body/mind division perpetrated by Western religions, there were many economic and political stirrings in eighteenth- and nineteenth-century Europe that contributed greatly to our present-day body prejudice. The rise of the middle class, or bourgeoisie, after the French Revolution created a repressive morality. Since this middle class believed that sexual and other excesses had contributed to the degeneration of the aristocracy, and that sexual degradation was prevalent among the poor, they were anxious to find ways to avoid the moral corruption that they imagined permeated the upper and lower classes. Therefore, a middle-class morality developed, which emphasized "self-reliance," "self-control" and "love of work," to quote Stephen Kern in *Anatomy and Destiny*.

This stress on bodily control and the importance of work became even more pronounced during the Industrial Revolution and the rise of capitalism in the nineteenth century. As industry flourished, the body came to be seen more as a mechanism for producing goods than as a source of pleasure. For a human being to be an efficient unit of production, it was important that he not squander his energies on activities other than work. Capital was to be reinvested for future profit, not spent on immediate pleasure. The same philosophy was applied to a person's emotions— particularly strong ones, such as anger, grief, joy, and sexuality. These were not to be spent rashly, and it was no accident that orgasms came to be referred to as "spending."

The harshest expression of this restriction on the needs of the body occurred in Victorian England and in the American Colonies, when the human body in its entirety became a taboo. Even the innocent (non-sexual) parts were hidden. It is reported that those symbols of romance, poets Elizabeth Barrett Browning and her husband, Robert, never once saw each other naked. Bodies were viewed as a source of temptation and sin. The Victorians believed that the sight of a female body or a part of it—even an ankle or an arm—could produce distracting and unwholesome sexual excitement which would leave men unable to concentrate on more important matters, like work. During the Victorian age, legs were rarely seen and were not even referred to by name; the discreet word "limb" was used. (There is a famous—and true—story of a headmistress of a New England woman's seminary who was so concerned about the provocative nature of any kind of leg that she covered the legs of a piano with four little pantalettes.) This daintiness was even extended to the animal world: a chicken leg became "dark meat" and a chicken breast, "white meat."

The bodies of women were covered literally from head to foot. The average woman wore layers of petticoats, a floor-length skirt (later in the century, with a bustle), a blouse with long sleeves and a high collar (except on formal occasions), a bonnet that completely covered her head, and frequently a shawl to further conceal her upper body. Even a lady's hands were hidden. An 1840 Victorian ladies' journal advised that "Gloves are always graceful for a lady in the house except at meals." And some women did not appear at the table "barehanded." They wore fingerless mittens.

A woman's body was not only obscured, it was distorted with one of the most uncomfortable articles of clothing ever invented—the corset. The results of a lifetime of corset wearing were appalling. Not only were women physically unable to exercise, they frequently could not even lean back in a chair without great discomfort. Since the wearers could take only short and shallow breaths, they were subject to frequent dizziness and fainting. The squeezing of their kidneys and bladders produced urinary disorders, constipation was a common malady, and the displacement and distortion of their reproductive organs caused miscarriages and painful and dangerous childbirth. When they removed their corsets, their naked bodies were an unlovely sight. The permanent disfigurements incurred might include a curved spine, lax stomach muscles, protruding buttocks, and black-and-blue bruises.

No matter how disfiguring they were, corsets were rarely removed. Uncorseted women were regarded as "vessels of sin." Women were encouraged to wear special corsets at night. They could even purchase special summer corsets which were guaranteed rustproof in case the wearer went swimming.

Men's bodies were also physically restricted, with narrow trousers, tight jackets, shirts that were stiff with starch, high collars that almost caused strangulation, high hats and, of course, long underwear. Corsets were fashionable for men for a time, a craze started by military officers who, in their gentleman's clubs, used to discuss the effectiveness of various types of corsets as earnestly as battlefield strategy.

Children fared no better. Their clothing was often a replica of adult fashions and just as uncomfortable. Little girls wore shorter skirts than their mothers, but the length depended on their age. A chart of the time shows the proper length for girls' skirts—somewhere below the knee at age four and descending to the shoe by puberty. Even little girls wore stockings and sometimes their undeveloped bodies were securely confined in a junior corset.

Bodies, including children's bodies, were considered essentially *sexual*, and the Victorians thought that sex was at best a necessary evil for propagating succeeding generations. Normal women were not expected to have sexual feelings, much less orgasms. Indeed, it was thought that a woman who did have orgasms might become infertile. Even the secretions of the Bartholin gland, which make a woman's genitals moist during intercourse, were thought to be abnormal and a sign that a woman was "lascivious." Manifestations of female sexuality, in the marriage bed or even through masturbation, could bring about repressive countermeasures. In the nineteenth century, doctors sometimes resorted to the surgical removal of the clitoris to cure women who masturbated "excessively."

Under these circumstances, few married couples were ever able to achieve a pleasurable or guilt-free sex life. Most women knew nothing about their own bodies, and the little information some women might have gotten from doctors was likely to be erroneous, for the knowledge medical men imparted about female sexuality was marked by their own prejudices and their lack of opportunity to learn about women's bodies. Doctors of that period, because they were only able to observe the bodies of corset-deformed women, believed that women breathed differently from men—i.e., only from the thorax. In addition, "modesty" prevented many women from going to a doctor who inevitably would be male. In fact, part of the motivation behind Elizabeth Blackwell's becoming the first woman doctor in America was her watching a woman friend die rather than let a male doctor treat her.

The attitudes toward male biology weren't any more enlightened. Men were taught that normal nocturnal emissions were dangerous and, if not controlled, would lead to a disease called spermatorrhea (involuntary discharge of semen while awake or asleep). This so-called disease was thought to be caused by squandering one's sexual energies, and so some husbands, on the advice of certain marriage manuals, restricted themselves to one orgasm a week. It is unlikely that his orgasm was shared by his wife, since few husbands had any knowledge of the sexual techniques that might arouse a woman. Indeed, they had no reason to learn such techniques since woman was not thought capable or desirous of orgasms. Her sole function as a sexual partner was to submit to her husband and bear him children. Single people, of course, weren't supposed to have a sex life.

Parents constantly watched their children (particularly sons) to make sure they didn't practice the dreaded "solitary vice." Children were prohibited from lingering in bed after they woke up, eating spicy foods, wearing clothing tight enough to rub against their genitals, or getting constipated, because all these things were thought to contribute to sexual arousal, which could lead to masturbation. If a child were found to be masturbating in defiance of all these precautions, he might be forced to wear a corset with a metal cup over his genitals, to have ice applied to his genitals at night, or to have his hands tied to the bedposts while he slept. He might even be forced to wear a metal ring around his penis which, if he started having an erection, would make him acutely uncomfortable.

Quite obviously people were not supposed to enjoy their bodies or sex. Nature, it was held, provided an appropriate punishment for those who did—in the form of venereal disease, particularly syphilis. Syphilis, as Stephen Kern points out in *Anatomy and Destiny*, "was an ideal Protestant disease, as well as an ironically Victorian disease. One transgression, a single sexual contact, could lead to a lifetime of suffering. There was no way of knowing for certain if one had been contaminated." The prevalent treatment during the latter part of the century was mercury, which supposedly raised the body's temperature and burned out the syphilis-causing bacterium, the spirochete. The price a person paid for this treatment was nausea and dizziness, black gums and loosened teeth, and the spitting out of up to a pint of saliva a day. These "wages of sin" seemed reason enough to support Victorian sexual morality; abstinence was the only reliable preventative of a disease for which the cure was both unsure and highly unpleasant.

THE VICTORIAN LEGACY

Superficially it may appear that we are rid of the Victorian body taboos. Many believe that we have gone too far in the direction of body display, sexual freedom, and the pursuit of bodily pleasure. Popular magazines feature pictures of nude males and females, in full frontal glory. Critically acclaimed movies portray nudity, urination, and explicit sex acts. Television documentaries explore subjects such as homosexuality and prostitution. And gatherings of men and women on almost every social level discuss the formerly "forbidden" subject of sex, if only in the form of "dirty jokes."

However, much of today's behavior is not so much a sign of real body liberation as it is a sign of rebellion against the past. Like children writing four-letter words on fences, people delight in verbally defying convention with talk of things that were, not so very long ago, taboo. But such conversation does not have the matter-of-fact tone of people who are comfortable with either the words they are using or their bodies. When it comes to everyday behavior, the naked human body is still pretty much off-limits. The very men and women who so liberally sprinkle their cocktail-party conversation with four-letter words would still be terribly embarrassed to be seen without clothes at an all-nude beach. Even today, unless you frequent "topless" bars (where only beautiful naked people are on display) or are in the field of health care, the only naked body you are apt to see is your sexual partner's.

The following is a questionnaire that can help you discover whether any remnants of Victorianism are preventing you from fully accepting and enjoying your body. Consider the B and C parts of the questions most carefully. These will give you some insights into your attitudes about your body and its functions.

There are no right or wrong answers to the questions. This is simply a consciousness-raising questionnaire. You should not assume that unless you can use all the terms and act in all the ways listed above that there is something wrong with you. However, it pays to take a look at some attitudes you may have taken for granted or avoided thinking about until now. If you can't say certain words—*ever*—or if it upsets you even to think about certain behaviors, you might want to free-up your thinking by examining just why these things disturb you.

Body Attitude Questionnaire

1. A. What do you usually say to a group of people when you leave the room to urinate?
(1) Nothing at all.
(2) Excuse me.
(3) I have to make a telephone call.
(4) I have to go to the bathroom, john, ladies' room (or some other euphemism).
(5) I have to go to the toilet.
B. What do you think of people who make the sort of statements you wouldn't make? Are you embarrassed? Why?

2. A. Which kinds of words for excretory products are you uncomfortable with?

(1) Euphemisms—number one, tinkle, number two, B.M., etc.
(2) Scientific terms—urine, feces, etc.
(3) Earthy terms—piss, shit, etc.
B. What about those terms makes you uncomfortable?
C. What words for excretory products do you feel perfectly comfortable using in public?

3. A. Which kinds of words for sexual parts and activities are you uncomfortable with?
(1) Euphemisms—private parts, "down there," making love, etc.
(2) Scientific terms—genitalia, penis, vagina, sexual intercourse, etc.
(3) Earthy terms—pussy, screw, etc.
B. What about those terms makes you uncomfortable?
C. What words for sexual parts and activities do you feel perfectly comfortable using in public?

4. A. In how many of the following situations would you be comfortable without clothing?
(1) In your doctor's examining room.
(2) In bed with your sexual partner.
(3) In a room with your children.
(4) Swimming.
(5) Getting a professional massage.
(6) In a locker room or dressing room with members of the same sex.
(7) At a nude camp or on a nude beach.
(8) In a sauna, jacuzzi or hot-tub with friends of both sexes.
B. In the situations where you would be uncomfortable, what are the beliefs or assumptions that would make you that way?

5. A. Which of these areas would you scratch in public if you felt the need? Your nose, arm, calf, thigh, foot, breast, buttocks, pubic area?
B. Why would you not scratch the other areas?
C. What would you think of someone who, in public, scratched or touched the body areas that you would

avoid? (E.g., they are vulgar, uninhibited, untrained, absent-minded.)
6. A. Would you feel embarrassed or guilty if friends or acquaintances saw you:
   (1) Looking through magazines that feature nude photos?
   (2) Going into a "topless" bar?
   (3) Going into an "adult" bookstore.
   (4) Browsing through sex manuals in a bookstore?
   (5) Buying contraceptives at a drugstore?
   (6) Going into an X-rated movie?
   or if they heard that you:
   (7) Went to a nude beach or camp?
   (8) Went to a sex clinic?
   (9) Joined a massage class?
   B. What do you suppose they would think about you?
   C. What would you think of someone else who did these things?
7. A. What are your reactions to women whose nipples can be seen through their clothes or whose breasts jiggle as they walk, or to men whose pants are so tight, the outline of their penises can be seen?
   B. Do you judge them as liberated, exhibitionistic, lewd, sexually available?

The Victorian legacy—the inheritance that prevents us from appreciating the naturalness of the human body and its functions—still lives on in all of us to some degree. While most people have freed themselves from a number of the body-disparaging attitudes of our cultural past, it is impossible to live in this society and not have at least some negative feelings about certain parts and certain functions of the body.

Chapter 3
Taking Charge of Your Body and Yourself

> We need to get away from the assumption that there is a *healer* up there and I am a *healee*, and the attitude that says, "Do something, fix me," as if a person were a car or a typewriter.
>
> Patricia Phillips, M.S.W.,
> Community Services Coordinator,
> Holistic Health Center, Los Angeles, California

Perhaps by now you are saying, "So what if I judge others by the way they look? So what if my feelings about my body aren't as positive as they could be? So what if I have some Victorian attitudes about sex? Such attitudes can't kill me. I've gotten along just fine so far and there are more important things in life to worry about than how I feel about bodies—mine or anybody else's."

If we've just quoted you, you're dead wrong. Body prejudice can kill you—in slow degrees perhaps—but it can kill you just the same. Lack of respect for the body and proper health care may well be the major causes of poor health in this country. If you are ashamed of your appearance or disgusted by some of your bodily functions you may fail to give your body the kind of day-to-day maintenance it requires. On the other hand, if you accept your body and appreciate the wonder and complexity of its functions, you will be receptive to learning more about the best ways to care for yourself.

THE RISKS OF BODY PREJUDICE

Let's take a look at the ways body prejudice may be depriving you of pleasure, shortening your life, and robbing you of energy.

Body prejudice leads to body avoidance. Embarrassment or shame about your body can keep you either from examining yourself or from going to the doctor to be examined, or both. A woman who is uncomfortable with the size, shape, or function of her breasts is not likely to give herself the recommended monthly breast exams. Because of her avoidance of looking at, touching, or examining her body, she may fail to notice a lump that could be malignant (and fatal, without medical care). A man who is uncomfortable about his genitals may ignore a sexual dysfunction that could be a symptom of prostate trouble. People who avoid looking at or thinking about their sexual organs generally fail to examine and care for themselves in ways that could prevent problems from developing, in addition to ignoring symptoms of dysfunction for potentially dangerously long periods.

Overweight people, in particular, may put off going to the doctor in the hope that they will lose weight before having to face the dreaded weigh-in. This delay can lead to heart attacks, strokes, diabetes, or other diseases that might have been alleviated or prevented had the doctor been able to discover and treat the symptoms earlier.

Body avoidance leads to body ignorance. Although our body is our primary natural resource—the source and distributor of our energy and joy—we are amazingly ignorant about it. Because we see countless bodies every day and because our body's optimum functioning is of vital importance to everything we do (from nursing our babies to performing well at our jobs), you'd think that bodies would intrigue every one of us. But the only people in our culture who concern themselves with studying bodies are in the field of medicine—researchers, doctors, nurses, and so forth. And their main concern is with the discovery and treatment of disease rather than with the study and promotion of human well-being. Despite their training, doctors, too, are victims of a kind of body ignorance that comes from body avoidance. They seem to pay as little attention to the care of their own bodies as the rest of us do. As a group, their health is no better than the rest of the population's.

As for most of us, except when we are injured or ill we are more concerned with the machines we use than with our bodies. Chances are, you have more respect for the intricate workings of your hi-fi or electronic calculator than you do for the workings of your nervous system. Chances are, you pay more attention to the functioning of your garbage disposal and washing machine than to that of your colon and kidneys. You may know more about Liz Taylor's love life than about the physiological factors that concern your own.

Curiosity, concern, and knowledge are all necessary for proper health care. Although it is customary to pay lip service to the wisdom of following good health habits, few people do. Here are seven guidelines that Dr. Lester Breslow, Dean of UCLA's School of Public Health, has found to be correlated with long, healthy lives:

1. No smoking.
2. Moderate drinking.
3. Seven or eight hours of sleep each night.
4. Regular meals with no snacks in between.
5. Breakfast every day.
6. Moderate, regular exercise.
7. Maintenance of normal weight.

Ignorance of your body's health needs is costly. Dr. Breslow studied groups of adults who followed the health guidelines listed above and found that the health of a person having these seven habits was better than that of a person having six, six better than five, and so on. A man of 45, for example, who has six or seven of these good health-habits is likely to live 11½ years longer than a man of 45 who has only three or fewer good health-habits.

Ignorance of what is good for one's body does not stem from a lack of available knowledge. Health-care information is abundant—in books, in classes, from one's doctor, and some is widely disseminated by the mass media. However, people who don't take pride in their bodies don't take notice of information about body care.

Body ignorance leads to body neglect. No scientific treatise is necessary to point up the body neglect in our society. There is evidence all around us that the most popular lifestyle today is one of body neglect. Let's take a look at how, everyday, the majority of people neglect their health, through ignorance or inaction, ignoring the seven basic health rules we listed earlier.

To start with, cigarette smoking is more than a bad habit; it is the number-one threat to the health of this country, according to the U.S. surgeon-general. Yet, in spite of the warnings of the surgeon-general, the American Cancer Society, and heart and lung specialists, some 53 million Americans smoked 607 billion cigarettes in 1975. Some people have gotten the message that cigarette smoking is harmful to their health; the percentage of men and women between the ages of 25-54 who smoke has dropped (some older smokers probably had begun to feel the ill effects on their bodies). However, one million young people each year begin the smoking habit and the percentage of teenage girls who smoke has increased. Young people seem more likely to copy the body-neglect lifestyle of their elders than to heed warnings about negative consequences on their health.

Drinking only moderately, the second basic health habit, is another thing both young people and adults find difficult to do. Young people make up half a million of the estimated ten million alcoholics in this country. Despite the widely publicized information about the harmful effects of excessive alcohol, despite the families broken up, children abused, careers destroyed, and accidents caused by people who can't seem to use alcohol moderately, and despite the economic hardships of recent years (inflation, recession, unemployment), the consumption of alcohol has increased considerably in the last ten years. Two-thirds of all adults drink. Alcohol (the major addictive drug sold legally without prescription in this country) is served at everything from baby showers to business meetings. Many find it easier to have a cocktail to slow down after work than to meditate or exercise. It seems easier to have a drink after a fight with one's spouse or boss than to try to resolve the conflict or work off the tension in other ways; it seems easier to drink to dull the stresses of life than to cope with them in more healthful ways—easier, that is, on everything but the body.

Third, many people do not get enough sleep—one of the body's most basic needs. With some, it is a matter of choice. They have chosen to stay up to watch the late, late show or to go to parties or to moonlight on an extra job to make more money. For others, lack of sleep is involuntary. Because of worries or stress or bad diet or lack of exercise—in short, because of body neglect—they are unable to fall asleep easily or to get a full night's sleep. Rather than examine their lives, they try to knock out their neglected bodies with alcohol, sleeping pills, marijuana, tranquilizers, or whatever else they think will work.

Most people do not eat properly, defying the fourth and fifth rules for good health, and defying the fact that, in many ways, "you are what you eat." Studies of the eating patterns of the American family indicate few families regularly sit down and eat together. Instead of having a good breakfast— the most important meal of the day—many skip this meal entirely or grab a snack on the run. Instead of having regular meals with no snacks in-between, snacking continues all day long—colas, French fries, doughnuts, hot dogs, potato chips, milk shakes, cookies, cakes, and candies. Hit-and-run snacking instead of regular sit-down meals might not be so bad if the snacks were nutritious, but many of them shouldn't even be described as food. Most consist either largely or entirely of "empty" calories (i.e., those deficient in energy-building nutrients). "Snacks" are often sugar-filled or coated, highly spiced or salted, and contain chemical additives. Yet people continue buying readily available junk food, easily prepared instant foods rather than body-building fresh foods, and few protest the addition to their foods of substances that may be downright dangerous to their health. Could the evidence for body neglect as an American way of life be more obvious?

Besides poor eating habits, another commonly neglected principle is moderate and regular exercise, rule number six of good health. An effective exercise program includes some of each of the three forms of exercise a body needs—stretching, toning, and strengthening. Though we see many more joggers, tennis players, and skiers than we used to, much of what we see is short-lived resolutions and impulsive trend following, rather than a concern for the welfare of the body. The average American either doesn't exercise at all, exercises sporadically ("weekend athletes"), or doesn't give his body the proper balance of exercise. This sort of exercising can be more punishing than beneficial.

All of the forms of neglect that we have been talking about result in bodies that don't feel as good as they should, look as good as they should, or function as well as they should. And these bodies are frequently overweight, ignoring our seventh principle of good health. Some authorities estimate at least one-fourth of all Americans are overweight. Toting around all that extra weight is hard on the body, particularly the heart. People who carry excess weight have a much greater likelihood of finding themselves with high blood pressure or diabetes. Control of one's diet—in terms of better nutrition and weight control—is recommended by the American Heart Association for reducing the risk of a cardiovascular disease (high blood pressure, heart attack, stroke, atherosclerosis, among others). These diseases affect 29 million Americans and kill one million a year—making cardiovascular diseases the number-one cause of death in this country.

Everyone has an excuse for body neglect—not enough time, not enough money, not enough energy—but the real cause is a value system that underrates body care. Body prejudice, body avoidance, body ignorance, and a lifestyle that not only encourages but is based on body neglect can only lead to poor health.

Body neglect leads to ill-health. As you may have realized by now, the chronic ill-health that many suffer does not stem from a lack of money spent on health care. In 1975, for example, close to 10 percent of the gross national product was devoted to medical care. But these statistics don't tell the story—the money hasn't resulted in a nation of people who feel good. Most of the money was spent by people who had neglected their bodies to the point that they became sick and had to receive medical treatment or be hospitalized; little was spent on keeping well.

Numerous books have appeared recently, filled with charts and statistics that point out the deplorable state of the health of the average American. While some lay the blame on the doorstep of organized medicine, and others blame the lack of controls on the food industry, and still others cite the declining quality of the environment, all agree that Americans aren't very healthy. You don't need to read it in a book; you can see it with your own eyes. Walk along a busy street, go to a supermarket, a railway station, or any other public place where people gather and you'll see the signs of poor health all around you—eyes that lack sparkle; shoulders that droop; a stiff or lagging walk that shows pain, stress, or chronic fatigue; a body that is out of alignment; unhealthy looking skin, hair, and teeth. It has almost become a new social ritual of "one-upmanship" to compare health notes to see who has felt the worst for the longest time.

Many people who are not technically "sick" in the way we usually define sickness in our society—that is, having symptoms of a disease or being under a doctor's care—don't realize they aren't healthy because they have no standards of comparison; they don't know what it is like to feel good. Those people who feel nervous, tired, and harried, lacking in zest and ambition, think it can't be helped, that their job or the problems of daily living (or something else they can do nothing about) is causing their discomfort. Chances are, most will drag on, not really ill but *un*well all of their lives—unless they reach a crisis and need medical attention or hospitalization. Even then, though their major symptoms may be treated, they'll probably go right back to the lifestyle that caused their health to break down.

LISTENING—AND RESPONDING—TO YOUR BODY MESSAGES

One reason many people are able to ignore their ill-health is that they have lost much of their body awareness—the ability to experience bodily sensations consciously, both those caused by physiological processes (e.g., food in the stomach) and those caused by emotional reactions (e.g., butterflies in the stomach). They are oblivious to body signals that could tell them what is happening in their bodies—of muscle contractions, stomach rumblings, rapid heart beats—and to the fact that they flush, shiver, or sweat in response to certain emotional stimuli. Although our language is full of expressions that show the countless ways our bodies communicate with us ("I feel it in my bones"; "He is a pain in the neck"; "My skin is crawling"), people growing up in a society that considers the body's needs less important than the Gross National Product have lost much of their ability to hear these messages.

Babies and little children pay attention to these messages and respond to them. They let others know when they need to eat, go to the toilet, run around, or go to sleep. However, as you learn appropriate social responses to your body messages (that you can't eat whenever you want to; that you have to control your excretory functions; that it isn't okay to have a tantrum in public), you also learn to suppress your awareness of some body sensations. It is not necessarily harmful to respond to body messages in socially approved ways but it is harmful to block your awareness so much that you don't know what is going on inside you. It is harmful to have to depend on the clock or social customs to tell you when you should eat, sleep, make love, or feel pain.

Some consider it an advantage to be unaware of bodily sensations, particularly those they consider unpleasant. Some boast that nothing bothers them—that they never have any aches or pains or, if they do, they don't "give in" to them. Being proud that you can't feel discomfort or can ignore it makes as much sense as training yourself not to smell smoke when there is something burning or to resist the impulse to investigate its source. Training yourself not to respond to something inside your body (chest pains, arm numbness) or outside your body (eye-burning smog, jet plane roar, overtly antagonistic people) can't help you get rid of the irritation. The truth is, what you don't know *can* hurt you.

Others who are painfully aware of some unpleasant body messages—a headache that strikes every night, chronic indigestion, or persistent neck tension—try hard to silence them with pills. Whether they think chronic aches and pains are natural (since they're widespread), or they believe their daily tasks are too important to be interrupted by visiting the doctor, or they find it distasteful to investigate the underlying sources of their discomfort, the result is that they suppress this important information their body is giving them with drugs. The causes, however, remain untouched.

Despite the media's alarm over illicit drugs, most of us in this country are pill-poppers. Fifty to 80 percent of the adult population take a prescribed drug nearly once a day. Just think of how many people you know who can't deal with daily stress without tranquilizers; who can't get to sleep without sleeping pills; who have a medicine cabinet chock full of palliatives for frequent bouts with headaches, colds, flu, constipation; or who keep antacid tablets in their nightstand for midnight heartburn and indigestion?

The medical profession aids and abets our pill-popping habits. When a patient complains of listlessness and other symptoms of chronic ill-health, the doctor, unable to find anything clinically wrong, often prescribes tranquilizers and advises the patient to "stop worrying," "slow down," and "roll with the punches." Relying on drugs to relieve symptoms instead of discovering and dealing with the underlying causes of sickness and chronic ill-health has reached epidemic proportions. And all of this is but another symptom of poor health caused by body neglect.

THE SATISFACTIONS OF BODY ACCEPTANCE

Body acceptance leads to body exploration. Good health starts with body acceptance, the opposite of body prejudice. You will not be as healthy as you can be until you fully accept your body—until you recognize that your body, just as it is, is worthwhile. This is something you will learn to do as you read this book and follow its suggestions.

It is ironic that while our society has encouraged the careful, scientific, and joyful exploration of other miracles of nature—Mount Everest, the moon, and the ocean floor—it has not encouraged the careful, scientific, and joyful exploration of the greatest miracle, the human body. When you begin to look at your body with the appreciation it deserves, you will discover the pleasure of exploring terrain previously unknown to you. As you explore it, you will find it more and more fascinating.

If you have never stood in front of a mirror, looked yourself over front and back, and then carefully explored, touching yourself from head to toe, this is the time to do it. If you have done it before, this is the time to do it again, and to start doing it regularly. Good health requires that you examine your body every day to stay aware of its constant changes. A good time to do this is as you dry off after your bath or shower or as you get dressed in the morning.

Body exploration leads to body knowledge. As your interest in exploring your body increases, you will probably develop a curiosity about your own anatomy and physiology. These subjects, generally left to scientists in our body-prejudiced society, can be fascinating to everyone. In addition, information about how a normal, healthy body functions can alert you to any potential problems in your own.

What could be more interesting than learning what makes you tick? Understanding how a human being's circulatory system works—what blood is made of, what it does, and how it gets where it needs to go—or learning the names and locations, and functions of the endocrine glands—how the hormones they secrete affect you at various ages and emotional stages—is no more difficult than teaching yourself astrology. And your physiology is likely to have more effect on your life than the positions of the sun and the moon and the stars. (Some good books to increase your body knowledge are listed in the bibliography.)

Medical books generalize about "normal" and "average" people. But there is no such thing as "typical." Though we all know that no two people—not even identical twins—look exactly alike, it may come as a surprise to discover that no two bodies function exactly alike either. Your temperature may consistently run a degree or more higher or lower than the "normal" 98.6° F.; a nutritive fruit for most people could give you hives; a sedative may act as a stimulant in your body; or a simple bee sting could be deadly to you.

By combining your own body examination with factual information, you'll be able to tell which bodily changes are within normal limits and which could be the first signs of an abnormal condition. If you notice such things as skin that becomes oilier or drier than usual, moles that change color or size, glands that seem swollen, hair growth in unusual areas, or changes in sexual organs, point them out to your doctor. Body knowledge and awareness can help you prevent problems from becoming serious.

Body knowledge leads to body care. Bookstores are loaded with books on nutrition, exercise, and diet, which can help you set up a good health-care regimen. Such a plan, however, must be custom-made to suit your needs—both physical needs and those fitting your particular lifestyle.

To help with this task, we suggest you keep a "body calendar"—one that has large blanks for each day, so that you can jot down significant facts about your body. Keep the calendar where it will be readily available (maybe on the inside of your medicine cabinet). Record such things as weight, menstrual cycle, allergic reactions, changes in bowel patterns, eating habits, unusual pains or symptoms, energy level, sexual interest, and anything else that could make your body feel good or bad. Record events that affect how you feel, what you eat or drink, your emotional reactions, and all medications that you take. (A sample calendar is provided on the opposite page.)

Keeping a body calendar will make it easy to relate what is going on in your life to how good or bad you feel. If you pay careful attention to your lifestyle and your body reactions, you will certainly discover connections. For example, migraine headaches and allergic reactions can sometimes be brought on by certain foods, chemical substances, or by a phone call from someone who upsets you.

Dr. Marilynn Pratt, physician, psychotherapist, and director of the Women's Institute in Los Angeles, California, believes a body calendar can be a useful diagnostic aid to your physician: "Patients who keep such a calendar are much more helpful in providing the information a doctor needs to make an accurate diagnosis, and thus when they become ill, they don't have to stay that way for so long."

Body care leads to good health and enjoyment. The kind of good health we are talking about means experiencing most of the time a sense of aliveness, awareness, and pleasure. This can happen only when you sense yourself as a complex entity—body and mind—constantly changing and in constant

TAKING CHARGE OF YOUR BODY AND YOURSELF

Body Calendar

Sunday	Monday	Tuesday	Wednesday	Thursday	Friday	Saturday
	1 weight 133 lbs. (2 lbs. up from last month)	2 irritable, tired; quarrel with John	3 insomnia, headache; took 2 aspirins	4 menstruating—cramps	5 menstruating; had pizza at Mother's	6 menstruating; diarrhea
7 menstruating; diarrhea	8 menstruating; bicycled—felt good	9 ate lunch in park with Sue—relaxing	10 in charge of PTA dinner—nothing went right; nervous; ate too much	11 fasted all day; stomachache; took antacid pills	12 examined breasts—O.K.; went dancing with John	13 cleaned house; tired but relaxed
14 went on 5-mile hike in mountains with family—great!	15 tried new low-calorie recipes	16 body feels better, filled but not overstuffed	17 played volleyball	18 have swollen arm	19 dinner at new French restaurant—ate snails for first time	20 have rash on hands and face
21 rash worse—allergic to snails?	22 still have rash	23 went to doctor—poison oak causing rash (from hike in mountains?)	24 Jane called, quarrel on phone—she hung up—insomnia, sleeping pill	25 dental checkup O.K.—made appointment six months from now	26 pizza at mother's	27 diarrhea—maybe because of pizza?
28 took bicycle ride along river	29 muscles ache, but feel great	30 had lunch with John, in town—fun—feel good				
			1 weight—130 lbs. hurray!	2	3	4

interaction with your environment and with those who are around you.

The following statements, based on a list drawn up by Paul Dingwall, social worker and a director of the New Age Health Care Services in Santa Ana, California, are characteristic of someone who has achieved the kind of total (or holistic) health we are concerned with. How many statements apply to you?

1. I am relaxed and have a high level of energy.
2. I am free of pain and discomfort.
3. I enjoy processes that bring me pleasure more than self-punishing ones.
4. I have moderate weight.
5. I have moderate appetites (smoking, drinking, eating, working, gambling, etc.).
6. I have good recuperative powers; infection and inflammation rapidly disappear.
7. I have a high resistance to invasion by foreign organisms.
8. I have the ability to relax easily and sleep soundly.
9. I have a general good mood with only mild fluctuations; a sense of optimism.
10. I have a sense of overall order in my life and a sense of relatedness to others.

This list reflects a growing interest in expanding the definition of good health to include lifestyle and the expression of emotions as well as physical fitness. Many in the field of health care are now beginning to study healthy people, particularly those who are exceptionally healthy, instead of limiting their observations to those who are sick.

In a recent study conducted at the Langley Porter Neuropsychiatric Institute of San Francisco, exceptionally healthy persons were subjected to stress, and biofeedback devices were used to measure (by means of brain waves, muscle tension, heartbeat, and respiration patterns) the way the subjects' internal systems returned to normal afterwards. The results suggest that exceptionally healthy people are different in a basic and crucial way—they seem to have achieved a high level of mind-body integration.

MIND-BODY INTEGRATION AND THE NEW CONCEPTS OF HEALTH

Dr. Thomas Greening, psychotherapist and editor of the *Journal of Humanistic Psychology*, explains just what it means to have mind-body integration: "You cannot have an event going on in the mind without it also going on in the body—in the blood chemistry, neurophysiology, musculature." When a person is integrated in body and mind, his systems are synergistic (working together), and he doesn't dissipate his energy in conflicting tendencies or processes. There is no internal argument, no problem of his heart wanting one thing, his mind another.

When we see a person functioning this way, we often say, "they've got it all together," meaning all systems are "go." You've probably had this feeling at certain times in your life when you were totally concentrated on what you were doing and it came naturally, almost effortlessly. Maybe, if you are a teacher, it was a time when words you didn't know you knew poured forth freely and easily. Your ideas were new and clear. Your students heard and understood and were excited about what you said. You felt their excitement and more words poured out. It could have been a time when you were playing tennis or dancing or singing with a choir. It didn't matter how well you were doing compared to someone else. You were unstressed. You felt fulfilled by your own efforts.

At these times when you are in tune, unstressed, you feel healthy—and you are! The people with a high level of mind-body integration feel this sense of flow and excitement much of the time. Even they need help in staying this way. Others need help in order to feel this way more often. An integrated, flowing feeling is the philosophy of good health— the antithesis of "dis-ease"—underlying a new type of health care that is developing.

What It Means to Have Holistic Health

This new kind of health care is sometimes called the "new medicine," but is more often called "holistic health," "holistic medicine," or "holistic healing" because it is concerned with the whole person—all aspects of his body, mind, and life—not with only the part that is causing a problem.

Holistic medicine differs from traditional medicine in several respects. Traditional medicine, when confronted with someone who is in ill-health, looks for the germ or physiological malfunctioning assumed to be causing the problem and treats that and that alone. Traditional medicine has become so specialized that you practically have to diagnose your own problem before you know what kind of doctor to go to. On the other hand, holistic healers include not just medical doctors, but nurses, nutritionists, psychologists, masseurs, acupuncture specialists, yoga instructors, ministers, art and dance therapists, as well as some special kinds of body therapists we'll discuss in the next chapter.

These people frequently work as a team and look beyond the initial symptom for the underlying cause that is related to a person's lifestyle (which includes body care) and personality structure (which helps determine how well one copes with stress). Holistic healers pay attention to a person's environment—the amount of air, water, and noise pollution he is subject to, to his patterns of work and relaxation, to the amount of time he spends with others and by himself, to the amount of joy and pleasure in his life, and most of all, they pay attention to how he thinks and what he does when he is in a stressful situation.

There is a correlation between personality and such diseases as colitis, ulcers, hypertension, asthma, problems of the lower back, and heart disease. Indeed, a person's emotional conflicts may be an important factor in all disease— even cancer. Dr. Harold Stone, executive director of the Center for the Healing Arts in Los Angeles, points out there is extensive literature on the psychogenic (emotionally caused) origin of cancer, dating back hundreds of years: "We believe that the majority of illnesses, including cancer, occur because of the way a person lives his life—the way he thinks, feels, moves, his relationships with his parents, his sexuality, his spirituality, etc. When these elements get in some way out-of-balance or are disowned, locked-up, or imprisoned, a person becomes ill. Imprisoned energies cause illness."

If it sounds farfetched or mystical to talk in those terms, it is because we are accustomed to dividing the responsibility for ourselves among doctors, who take care of our bodies, and teachers, ministers, and others, who take care of our minds. Every time a person gets sick or is depressed or tired, there is something he needs and his body is expressing the need. Sometimes what the person needs is more attention from others and being sick gets it for him. Sometimes what he needs is a different job, one that nourishes his mind or spirit—illness will periodically take him away from his unsatisfactory job. Sometimes he needs time to rest and daydream—a high temperature will allow his mind time to float around in an altered state of consciousness. Sometimes he needs to give up sex because there is not enough caring that goes along with it. (The often repeated joke about wives who get headaches when they go to bed is no laughing matter, but an imbalance that should be looked into.)

You don't wait until you are sick to go to a holistic health center. All holistic health centers offer a variety of educational programs for people who are well. Though holistic healers are interested in curing illness, their basic thrust is with the prevention of future illness and the achievement and maintenance of a high level of "positive wellness."

No two holistic health centers are exactly alike. Each differs in what it offers and the direction it takes in working toward increased body-mind integration. For example, the Women's Institute and Health Center in Los Angeles, founded by Dr. Marilynn Pratt, general practitioner and psychotherapist, includes (in addition to the usual medical services available at a doctor's office) psychological services plus a wide variety of classes in such areas as yoga, dance, self-defense, reducing, sex education and general health education.

The Center for the Healing Arts, on the other hand, offers no general medical services, and focuses its classes on expanding consciousness and increasing personal awareness. In addition, it features a very unusual research center for cancer patients. In order to learn to deal with the part that stress has played in their illness, cancer patients participate in group and individual psychotherapy, attend weekly healing seminars, and are instructed in such self-healing procedures as breathing and relaxation techniques, yoga, meditation, and physical fitness. These activities do not take the place of medical treatment, but are in addition to whatever treatment the patient may be getting from his own physician.

At the Holistic Health Center in Los Angeles, although they have programs for arthritic patients and those suffering from cardio-vascular diseases, the outstanding feature is a "wellness program." Patrons are called clients, not patients, a term that eliminates the feeling you are turning over the control of your body to someone else. This center helps clients take a thorough look at themselves and their lifestyles in order to discover the areas in which they are functioning well, the areas that need to be changed, and particular health hazards to guard against. The initial assessment includes medical questionnaires and examinations, laboratory tests, an extensive lifestyle inventory, a thorough nutritional analysis, and numerous in-depth interviews. The client is assisted by a health-resource guide who works closely with him, explaining everything from the preliminary assessment phase to the final treatment. The resource guide works not only with the client but with a team of doctors, nurses, psychologists, social workers, art and dance therapists, exercise specialists, and massage experts, who formulate a program for enhancing the client's level of wellness. Clients' needs vary widely. While one person might require biofeedback, hormones, a high protein diet, and a vacation, another might need more iron and traces of zinc in his diet, vocational counseling, swimming, art therapy, and meditation.

However, no matter what form holistic health care takes, it stresses personal responsibility, insisting people learn to take charge of their own bodies. Pat Phillips, of the Holistic Health Center, says, "The center does not hover over clients or promise cures; instead, it insists clients take responsibility for what they need to make them feel good and enjoy life. This involves education and so people need to search and read and learn to evaluate. It doesn't mean that people need to become medical experts; it does mean that they need to be informed of the fact that they do have choices—and of just what these choices are. Therefore, it is important that they enter into a dialogue with whoever is going to participate in their health care and not just be a listener."

Though you do not need to become a medical expert in order to take charge of yourself and your body, you do need to become your own "body expert." The more you accept your body, the better prepared you are to take care of it in the ways necessary for achieving mind-body integration. The more you know your body—its feelings, its symptoms, its appearance—the better use you can make of experts in your life—your doctor, nutritionist, meditation teacher, tennis coach, exercise instructor, masseur, or therapist—as your consultants. However, you are in charge.

In addition, joining the Association for Humanistic Psychology or the Association for Holistic Medicine will keep you in touch with developments in this new area and help you maintain a holistic attitude.

Achieving holistic health, which also involves achieving mind-body integration, means more than the physical care of your body. You will have to lose some inhibitions that stem from body prejudices and which cause you to suppress strong emotions and limit your enjoyment of bodily pleasure. Unshed tears, pent-up resentments, unresolved conflicts, and unexpressed desires can kill you just as surely as the neglect of your nutritional needs or a lack of rest and relaxation.

In the next chapter we'll talk about some means for achieving open emotional expression and for acquiring stress-free ways of moving, standing, and sitting.

Chapter 4
Integrating Your
Mind and Body

> Since our deepest traumas are imbedded in our guts and muscles, to free ourselves we must free our bodies. Yet we are more than just bodies. We are minds and spirits, feelings and imaginings. And though the body speaks, it must always be the whole person to whom we listen.
>
> Ron Kurtz and Hector Prestera, M.D.
> *The Body Reveals: An Illustrated Guide*
> *to the Psychology of the Body*

The normal and natural way to express emotions is with our bodies. Look at a little boy who is hurt. His breathing changes, his body droops, his lips and jaw tremble, his chest, stomach, diaphragm, and throat muscles move, his eyes fill with tears, and he cries. Emotion is felt throughout his body and then discharged. He feels much better. But as he grows up society teaches him that tears are unmanly, that expressing emotions shows lack of control. He learns to suppress his tears. He uses a lot of energy to keep many muscles in his body absolutely still so they won't betray his feelings. If he continues to comply with the taboos against the bodily expression of emotions, eventually, like a robot, he won't even know when he has been hurt or is sad. He will have lost the ability to feel. He will be affected by life, but he will not respond. His unexpressed emotions will accumulate, causing internal pressure. They will be blocked in his body like a river behind a dam. Muscle patterns that hold his emotions in check will become a part of him, limiting his movements, making him rigid and ungraceful, keeping his body tense and full of stress, even changing its contours.

The blocking of feeling has a crippling effect, both physically and emotionally. Spontaneity and creativity are inhibited. Enthusiasm is lost. A person who consistently denies his feelings cannot possibly have the sort of mind-body integration that is basic to good health.

Some emotions such as anger, fear, pain, and grief are not pleasant, but we must learn to allow even these to flow unimpeded through our bodies. You can't turn off some feelings without turning off others. If you seldom or never discharge feelings you wish you didn't have, you will not be able to experience joy, to revel in sensations, to be comfortable with your sexuality, to be affectionate.

We do not suggest that being healthy, loving, and full of zest means always "giving in to your feelings," always expressing what you want, when you want it, no matter what the circumstances, no matter what the effect on other people. There is a difference between being in touch with your feelings and an immature need for instant gratification. When you are in touch with your feelings, you are better able to act in ways that are good both for yourself and others, able to act with responsibility based on knowledge.

BODY THERAPY LEADS TO BODY LIBERATION

To help people who block their feelings, a new type of therapy came into existence—body therapy. This therapy seeks to tap the power of the emotions in order to liberate the body. Body therapy consists of many therapies that can be grouped into two basic types: the *emotionally liberating* and the *physically liberating*.

The emotionally liberating therapies are aimed at releasing and redirecting the flow of strong emotions within the body. In the process, a person's appearance and movements may change. For example, as a person learns to release certain emotions, his facial expression may soften. He may no longer tense his jaw or tighten his facial muscles to keep from betraying involuntary signs of emotion. After a man who has long suppressed his sense of fear experiences and releases it, his walk may become more confident, his shoulders more relaxed. After a woman learns to feel her anger and to express it appropriately, she may stand straighter and look people in the eye. Releasing energy previously used to block feelings can result in better posture, easier breathing, more zest—better physical and emotional health.

The physically liberating therapies are designed to realign the body and help one move more freely. As a consequence, there is a release and redirection of considerable amounts of emotion. Physical activities affect the emotions. You may experience an emotional "charge" when you whack the tennis ball with extra vigor or kick your leg high into the air during an exercise routine. When you walk with your chest out and your head up, emotions are freed. By learning new tension-free ways of moving, feelings are also released—particularly joyful ones.

Before describing these activities, it is important to emphasize that "body therapy" is a convenient term for a variety of highly complex theories and methodologies that affect both body and mind. According to Dr. Thomas Greening, coordinator of a lecture series on the body therapies at UCLA: "Actually, there isn't any such thing as strictly 'body' therapy any more than there is such a thing as strictly 'psycho' therapy. You can't split the body from the psyche. What we are talking about are therapies which use the body and the physical experiencing of a person as entry into his whole being rather than using words or word images as is done in verbal therapy."

Body therapy is not a treatment for the "emotionally sick." It is basically a form of education for all of us reared in a body-prejudiced society. In fact, it is usually not realistic to categorize people as emotionally sick—all of us have problems coping with our emotions at times. All of us are in constantly changing states of body-mind integration, more or less in balance and always able to add to our education.

THE EMOTIONALLY LIBERATING THERAPIES

We will describe three kinds of emotionally liberating therapies: Reichian therapy, bioenergetics, and Radix education.

All derive from the work of Wilhelm Reich, the "father of body therapy."

Reichian Therapy

Reich, an Austrian physician, worked with Sigmund Freud, but came to question the psychoanalytic view of neuroses. In 1939 Reich came to the United States where he further developed his alternative theories of mental health. In his later years, some of his theories and methods (e.g., the "orgone box") were thought to be so bizarre that he was ostracized by most conventional psychiatric and psychological authorities. But his emphasis on how a person's emotional health was related to his capacity to experience orgasm was a valuable contribution to psychology. Reich proposed a form of therapy to improve one's ability to achieve sexual release (and so achieve general emotional health) that involved a nonerotic "laying-on of hands."

Though some of Reich's theories have been seriously misunderstood in the past, the truth of the idea that *the mind and body are one and must be treated as one* is presently acknowledged to be of tremendous importance and has had a large role in revolutionizing the way we treat ourselves and one another.

Reich believed that stress or neuroses become built into our bodies and that it is necessary to work with the body itself in order for the neuroses to be cured. As we grow up, we develop a pattern of chronic muscular tensions which Reich called "body armor." These tensions are real and observable; you can feel them; scientists can measure them with instruments. Observe how your own body behaves next time you are in an uncomfortable situation—when you are at your new boss' home for dinner, or when a neighbor unexpectedly drops in during a family argument. See if you are clamping your jaws, if your neck and shoulder muscles feel tight, if your stomach has knots. These signs mean you are trying to block out emotions.

We learn to develop body armor. A child learns to hold in his anger because he gets spanked if he admits he wants to hit his baby brother. He learns to inhibit physical affection when his hugs are rejected. Feelings that can't be expressed become locked in the body by chronic tension. In addition to developing chronic muscle tension, a person afraid of strong feeling may develop a habitual pattern of shallow breathing. Most of us unconsciously alter our breathing patterns when strong emotions are triggered—for example, we gasp or hold our breath when surprised or enraged.

Reich found that feelings could be unblocked by the deliberate alteration of breathing patterns—e.g., by breathing faster and more deeply. During therapy Reich applied pressure to the places that were "armored," facilitating the spontaneous release of held-in emotions. Through physical manipulation to remove chest armoring, breathing is permanently improved. Because of the discharge of strong emotions through crying, screaming, and swearing, the Reichian-based therapies can be noisy.

In addition to physical work with the body, there is an analysis of character traits and attitudes. Psychological as well as physical armor is broken down.

Today, those who follow Reich's teaching most closely—all of whom are medical doctors and most of whom are psychiatrists—call themselves medical orgone therapists, and orgonomy is a medical specialty. In Reichian therapy a patient usually lies on a couch in his underwear while the therapist sits next to him on a chair in order to better observe and work with his body.

Actor Orson Bean believes that the changes brought about in him during his three-and-a-half years of Reichian therapy with Dr. Ellsworth Baker (the man designated by Reich himself to be his training therapist) were profound.

The following selection from Bean's book, *Me and the Orgone*,* demonstrates some of the characteristic elements of Reichian therapy, i.e., the verbalization of immediate feelings, the deliberate alteration of breathing patterns, the spontaneous discharge of emotion and the relating of long suppressed feelings to significant past events.

> "You feel contemptuous of me?" [Baker asked.]
> "Well, I must, I suppose."
> "You suppose?"

---

*Reprinted with permission from "Me and the Orgone," by Orson Bean, copyright © 1971 by St. Martin's Press, Inc.

"All right, goddamnit, I *do*!"
"Feel what?"
"Contemptuous! Jesus!"
"What's the matter?"
"I *told* you what I felt."
"But I didn't feel it from you."
"All right, dammit, it's a lot of crap... lying here rolling my eyes around."
"Stick your finger down your throat," said Baker.
"What?" I said.
"Gag yourself."
"But I'll throw up all over your bed."
"If you want to you can," he said. "Just keep breathing while you do it."

I lay there breathing deeply and stuck my finger down my throat and gagged. Then I did it again.

"Keep breathing," said Baker. My lower lip began to tremble like a little kid's, tears began to run down my face and I began to bawl. I sobbed for five minutes as if my heart would break. Finally, the crying subsided.

"Did anything occur to you?" asked Baker.

"I thought about my mother and how much I loved her and how I felt like I could never reach her and I just felt hopeless and heartbroken," I said. "I felt like I was able to feel these things deeply for the first time since I was little, and it's such a relief to be able to cry and it isn't a lot of crap, I was just scared."

"Yes," he said. "It is frightening. You have a lot of anger to get out, a lot of hate and rage and then a lot of longing and a lot of love. Okay," he said, "I'll see you next time."

Through many of these unusual sessions, Bean got in touch with the "frightened child" part of his personality, as well as with other parts he had somehow lost contact with. By rediscovering these parts and integrating them into his personality he was able to become a healthier and more effective person. Bean founded an experimental school in New York, based on Reich's ideas, so that children would have an opportunity to grow up "unarmored"—learning to freely express their emotions and their humanity.

Bioenergetics

One brand of neo-Reichian therapy (therapy based on the concepts of Reich but differing in techniques used) is bioenergetics. In 1956 psychiatrist Alexander Lowen, one of Reich's best-known students and author of *Bioenergetics*, and his colleagues John C. Pierrakos and William B. Walling formed the Institute for Bioenergetic Analysis in New York City. Like Reich, Lowen considers his work therapeutic, but believes there are no cures—only a continuing process towards better and better health.

"Our bodies are our pasts," says Lowen. The overall appearance and functioning of our bodies—build, musculature and alignment, the way we move—depends to a considerable extent upon the emotional environment in which we were reared. How we were treated as children predisposes us to the build-up of certain muscular and psychological defenses.

Like Reich, Lowen believes mind and body are connected. Sometimes blood vessels contract in response to demeaning words; shoulders droop because of a longing for tenderness; spines stiffen from a feeling of too much responsibility. When these reactions become chronic, they interfere with fundamental physiological processes, such as blood flow, digestion, and biochemical reactions, which in turn influence such basic aspects of body build and appearance as the size and shape of the legs, the circumference of the waist, the way the head rests on the neck, the expression in the eyes.

These reactions also interfere with the flow of energy in our bodies and our ability to feel emotions. People have characteristic ways of defending (i.e., protecting) themselves against strong emotion—through behavior, thoughts, and muscles. Lowen has classified people into five basic personality types according to characteristic "defensive positions." But he stresses that while one may exhibit more characteristics of one type than another, no one exactly fits the stereotype. Consider the classifications not as a means of determining whether you are "abnormal," but as examples of the different ways people can and do react to their emotional environment.

These types are: (1) schizoid, (2) oral, (3) psychopath, (4) masochistic, (5) rigid.

1. The schizoid is a person lacking in feelings of self-worth. He tends to be withdrawn and unaware of what is going on either in himself or the world around him. His face lacks expression, he doesn't look you in the eye, his body parts don't seem to go together, and in many cases there is marked discrepancy between the upper and lower halves of his body.

2. The oral personality has a tendency to cling to others, to be unassertive, to have an extreme need to be held, supported, and taken care of. He is often tall and thin, with underdeveloped muscles, usually most noticeable in his arms and legs.

3. The psychopathic character type is overly concerned that others consider him important and has an extreme need to control everything and everybody either by bullying or seduction. The body of the psychopath may reflect how he gets his way with others. The upper half may be disproportionately heavy and overpowering, corresponding to the individual's blown-up image of himself. Or if he achieves power through seduction rather than force, his body may be more regular, but characterized by a hyperflexible back.

4. The masochist type suffers a great deal and whines and complains. But he remains submissive, doing little or nothing to prevent or stop his suffering. He often has a short, thick, muscular body, and a whipped-puppy type of posture.

5. The rigid character worries a great deal about being taken advantage of, used, or trapped. He is afraid to give in or reach out to others; he fears being considered weak. He holds his head high; his back is straight as a broomstick; his whole body is stiff.

Lowen originated a number of body positions that aid in the diagnosis of the blocks causing emotional stress, that "charge" the body with energy, that stimulate breathing. The main body position is the arch or bow. The patient is told to place his feet apart, turn his toes in a bit, bend his knees slightly, place both fists on his back just below the waist, and to arch his back like a bow drawn for action. When a person's body is in the bow or any of the so-called "stress" positions, a flow of energy develops and strong emotional reactions are triggered. When the body is in physical and emotional stress, its defenses against feeling go into operation and characteristic blocks can then be observed, felt, and broken through. The defenses are not destroyed but are made less controlling.

With the therapist's guidance, the patient, who is wearing a bathing suit, will read his own body to see what the automatic blocking of strong emotion has done to him. The therapist then helps him temporarily put aside his defenses, get in touch with his feelings, and reclaim parts of himself he has lost contact with. At times a person will be encouraged to shout words that evoke strong inner responses.

For example, a masochist type who tends to invite people to put all their problems on his back—and then, as a consequence, sees people as a burden—may be encouraged to repeat over and over, "Get off my back." Heavy emotional release—tears, rage, laughter, trembling—is often part of bioenergetics therapy. Such release is a sign that the defenses are being broken through and that energy is flowing freely throughout the body.

The goal of this new body therapy is to help people regain what Lowen calls their "primary nature," which is "the condition of being free, the state of being graceful, and the quality of being beautiful. Freedom, grace, and beauty are the natural attributes of every animal organism. Freedom is the absence of inner restraint to the flow of feeling, grace is the expression of this flow in movement, while beauty is a manifestation of the inner harmony such a flow engenders. They denote a healthy body and also, therefore, a healthy mind."

Radix Education

The Radix Institute in Santa Monica, California, was founded in 1960 by Dr. Charles Kelley, another of Reich's students. The objectives of this neo-Reichian therapy, Kelley explains, are educational: "We don't cure people of anything. What we will do is help them have an experience in which they make contact with their deepest feelings and become able to expand their capacity for feeling. Some people come in and they can't cry; their very ability to cry has been taken out of them. This is particularly true of men. Women are more likely to be unable to experience and express rage—this ability has been taken out of them in our society."

Kelley combines Reichian techniques with group dynamics, because, he believes, this combination lessens the tendency for clients to transfer feelings for past significant figures (such as parents) onto present significant figures such as therapists. Working in a group with four or five people makes it easier for the instructor to remain objective. In addition, a person may be triggered to release his own deep feelings by watching the work of others in the group.

Radix classes can vary from single-shot experiences (such as a weekend workshop) to on-going sessions. As with bioenergetics, Radix clients work in bathing suits so that the leader can watch breathing and muscle-tensing patterns and touch the stress-packed areas in ways to help release blocks to the flow of energy.

The highlight of a Radix session is an experience called the "intensive," during which a great deal of emotion is discharged. It is the most dramatic part of Radix education—the part people usually talk about. As a result, some people have the distorted view that the function of Radix education is to turn one's life into a series of emotional explosions. But clients do not wind up unable to control themselves, yelling at their bosses, crying over missed buses. Radix does not strip a person of his defenses. It helps him *use* his defenses more effectively and purposefully. Kelley says, "In doing Radix work we open the capacity to feel without destroying the capacity to block."

Reichian therapy, bioenergetics, and Radix education are only three of several kinds of emotionally liberating body therapies. Probably more kinds will emerge as holistic medicine becomes more widespread, making people realize how bodies, feelings, health, enjoyment of life, and productivity are all intertwined. (For references on body therapies, where you can find more information about them, and how you can locate a qualified body-therapist, see the lists at the end of the book.)

PHYSICALLY LIBERATING BODY THERAPIES

Our bodies are tilted and twisted in ways that force us to use excessive amounts of energy for routine activities. We have forgotten, if we ever knew, how free and light a graceful, well-aligned, well-functioning body can feel. We have also lost the full use of our sixth sense, the kinesthetic or body sense, which alerts us to pressures and tensions in the body, makes us aware of our gestures and movements, and helps us adapt to the weight of things we lift.

There are five factors that contribute to our having potbellies, pains in the back, or stiff joints.

1. *Man walks upright and not on all fours.* Our head is balanced on top of a long flexible stick—the spine. Because of the pull of gravity, it is easy for a person's body to get out of alignment. If, for example, something causes the upper part of the body to habitually bend forward—whether it is a whiplash or a chronic feeling of carrying the weight of the world on one's shoulders—the lower part of the body has to compensate by moving in the other direction. Otherwise, a person would fall flat on his face because of the downward pull of gravity.

2. *Our bodies literally get "molded" into shape by our parents while we are children.* As babies, with soft muscles, we can roll around freely, put our toes in our mouths, and contort our bodies in various ways. As we grow up, in addition to changing physically, we learn how we are to use our bodies. A little girl may learn to make "dainty" movements. A little boy may learn a sort of stiff-legged masculine strut that pleases his parents. As we develop our own particular style of standing, sitting, and moving, a sheet of connective tissue (fasciae) forms over the muscles, holding them in place. Ligaments and tendons adjust in length and bind bones and organs into position. In time, our body becomes "set."

3. *Our society places a high value on our not displaying our reactions.* Children are admonished: "Can't you ever sit still?" "Take it easy," "Don't talk with your hands." Small wonder our postures and movements become stiff, our ability to express ourselves with body movements becomes stifled.

4. *Our bodies are required to conform to the demands of a technological society.* We treat our bodies as if they were machines and try to get them to adapt to uncomfortable furniture, space limitations, rigid time schedules, and uncivilized work habits. Chairs, for example, come in hundreds of

shapes, but few fit the configuration of the human body. Our bodies have to adapt themselves to conform to the furniture of our society. On the other hand, in primitive or Eastern societies, where chairs are seldom or never used, it is easy for people to sit cross-legged on the ground or floor.

5. *We are taught to conform to our society's work ethic.* A six-year-old learning to write will hunch up his shoulders, tighten his face into a frown, and tense his entire body. He is developing a body-set that will carry into adulthood. Although the process of writing will eventually become easier, his body will "remember" the tension under which the skill was learned and will automatically slip into a "tension-set" whenever he writes. Tension will accompany the performance of any activity that was learned under tension—be it driving a car, mowing the lawn, or skiing.

The three physically liberating body therapies we are going to discuss—Rolfing, the Alexander technique, and the Feldenkrais method—have been designed to counteract these body-set problems. These therapies are not exercise classes. They are *psycho*-physical methods, acknowledging a mind-body unity: The mind will function better when the body feels good; the body will feel good when the mind functions well. This psycho-physical education aims at encouraging people to find pleasure in their bodies and teaching them how to consciously use their minds to prevent the reestablishment of painful or inhibiting body habits.

Rolfing

Though you may periodically have the wheels on your car realigned, it probably has never occurred to you that your body needs to be realigned, that you may need to be "rolfed." Rolfing, also called structural integration, is a method of intensive bodily manipulation. It is named after the woman who developed it, Dr. Ida Rolf, formerly an organic chemist with the Rockefeller Institute.

Rolfing is not something you can do yourself. It involves at least ten one-hour sessions and must be conducted by a therapist (rolfer) trained by the Rolf Institute in Boulder, Colorado. At each session, while the client lies undressed on a massage table, the therapist manipulates a particular part of the body. Indeed, the manipulation is so extensive that pictures taken at the beginning and end of each session reveal actual bodily changes.

For the five reasons stated previously everyone's body gets out of alignment to some degree; rolfing can correct this. Through the years, the connective tissue that holds organs in place and attaches bones to other bones and muscles to bones shrinks to accommodate the changing body—the body that gets shorter or hunches forward or tilts sideways. As the tissue shrinks, it also sticks to bones or muscles or other connective tissue to form adhesions. As a result, a person is not able to stand straight or move freely. Adhesions and shortened connective tissue literally lock a person into an awkward, uncomfortable, stressful position. Rolfing lengthens the connective tissue and frees the adhesions, making it possible for a person to stand up straight—to be correctly aligned.

Since the old adhesions have been in place a long time and since the connective tissue has to be stretched or pulled loose, rolfing can be a painful process, something people who have not been rolfed are quite concerned about. However, those who have been rolfed usually consider the benefits worth the pain. When the adhesions are broken loose, the connective tissue lengthened, the basic body lines properly organized, the body tends to move in a more flowing, graceful way that takes less energy.

Some people report that rolfing increases their ability to experience feeling in certain parts of their bodies, such as in the pelvic region. A result in these cases is that movements during sex become freer (overcoming an impairment perhaps due to having been taught that pelvic movement was vulgar). Some persons have also reported positive emotional changes—for example, an improved ability to handle anxiety. Indeed, some psychotherapists believe rolfing is a valuable adjunct to therapy, for it can bring out deep feelings suppressed since childhood.

The Alexander Technique

The Alexander technique's originator, F. M. Alexander, born in Australia in 1869, developed his theories when, as a Shakespearean actor, he found himself repeatedly losing his voice during his performances. Determined to discover what happened physically to bring this about, he set himself on a course of self-observation, carefully watching even his smallest movements in the mirror. He discovered that what caused him to lose his voice—and what controlled all of his movements—was the relationship of his head to his spine. When head and spine were out of proper alignment, all of his body movements were awkward and unnatural. He reasoned that correcting improper alignment required concentrating on the entire body at once, but emphasizing the head-spine relationship.

Like rolfing, the Alexander technique strives to bring the body back to its natural alignment. The student feels a new upwardness, lightness, and ease in his movements by eliminating the tensions caused by poor habits of posture and movement. However, its methods are quite different from rolfing. An Alexander therapist gives repeated instructions for autosuggestion, such as, "Let the neck be free," "Let the head go forward and up," "Let the back lengthen and widen." Simultaneously, the therapist moves his student's body in subtle ways. The Alexander movements are basically those of daily life—sitting, standing, walking, bending, lying down, etc. What one learns can be used to release the tension accompanying any activity—driving, playing tennis, ballet dancing, acting, or even playing a musical instrument.

The Alexander technique is currently a popular type of training in the theatrical world. It is also offered at the Institute of Rehabilitation Medicine in New York to patients suffering from such problems as low backache, pinched nerves, scoliosis (curvature of the spine), or tension. Educator John Dewey advocated the establishment of the Alexander technique in American public schools over fifty years ago, and some New York high school students now receive instruction.

The Feldenkrais Method

The physically liberating body system of exercise developed by Moshe Feldenkrais, an Israeli physicist, like the Alexander technique involves using the conscious control of the mind to help free the body. But it is unlike the Alexander technique in three important ways.

First, while an Alexander teacher works with one student at a time and uses his own hands to help teach the student new ways of moving, a Feldenkrais teacher works with a group of students. The students are told what to do and what to think, and then they practice on their own.

Second, while the Alexander technique focuses on helping people relearn tension-free ways of doing ordinary things, the Feldenkrais method focuses on helping people enlarge their repertoire of movements.

Third, while the Alexander lessons are conducted in essentially the same way for each person, the Feldenkrais method has over two thousand exercises, and a student may never do the same one twice.

The Feldenkrais method works by reestablishing the connections between the mind and the muscles that have been short-circuited by bad habits, tensions, and life-long conditioning. The exercises involve no stretching and straining, no trying to see how many push-ups you can do or how fast you can do them. Thus you never leave a session feeling stiff and sore. It is surprising what the body can do after only one Feldenkrais lesson involving slow, gentle, nonrepetitive movements.

At the first session a person is tested to determine what he can do with ease. For example, he might be asked to sit facing forward and, without moving his body, to turn his head to one side and see how far he can twist it *with ease*. He is next asked to do a very slow series of simple, easy exercises requiring no more effort than lifting a toothpick. Then he is told to test himself again—and he usually discovers his head can turn farther than before, farther than he ever thought possible.

Sometimes the student is asked to merely *think* through the exercises, and often the improvement is comparable to—or better than—what would have been accomplished if he had actually done them. How can thinking be the same as doing? Experiments have shown that even the thought of doing a movement causes activity in a muscle that can be recorded by special instruments. The mind, it seems, can take over much of the work that the body does, so the body does not need to push itself as hard. In most Feldenkrais lessons, however, both physical and mental sides are exercised so the student can be more aware of all the movements.

The benefits of both the Alexander and Feldenkrais methods (now being taught at universities, at dance and music schools, and in geriatric programs) are great. Judith Stransky, teacher of both methods and director of the American Center for the Alexander Technique in Santa Monica, says:

"The Alexander technique and the Feldenkrais method give to people a feeling of joy and ease with themselves. Although both methods use a different process, they utilize the same philosophy—no straining, effortlessness, subtle, gentle work, being kind to yourself and directing easily with the mind. The results are usually far beyond a person's conception of what he can feel like and how he can go through life. Some people say they now *float through life*. Sensitivity awareness is enormously heightened as a result of these methods. Often relationships improve and almost always pains and discomforts are relieved. And last, but not least, most students lose their self-consciousness and feelings of awkwardness or inferiority as a result of the great feeling of freedom that they have acquired."

The Alexander and Feldenkrais methods plus the other therapies we have discussed in this chapter have helped many people learn to free their bodies from some of the destructive inhibitions created by body prejudice, to achieve greater mind-body integration and, therefore, better holistic health. In the next chapter we'll discuss another form of therapy that can also help bring about these benefits by breaking down the taboos against seeing and touching bodies.

Chapter 5
Breaking the Seeing and Touching Taboo

> Touch
> is one of the basic languages
> of muscles, nerves, love.
> Mothers instinctively
> touch their children
> to comfort;
> hold them close to relax
> and reassure.
> To be held is support;
> to be touched is contact;
> to be touched sensitively
> is to be cared for.
>
> Bernard Gunther,
> *Sense Relaxation: Below Your Mind*

All bodies need to be looked at and touched with affection. Body acceptance and mind-body integration—the very basis of good health—cannot be achieved in isolation. Because body taboos put barriers between people, few of us ever get our fill of the vitally necessary physical and emotional nourishment that comes from loving body contact with others. We stand before a banquet table unable to eat.

Historically, when a need becomes great enough, a solution emerges to fill it. Because the Victorian practices of covering and denigrating bodies caused so much stress and unhappiness and sent people scurrying to psychotherapists, a type of interpersonal group experience evolved—nude therapy. This therapy, using the nude body as its major therapeutic tool, quickly breaks down some of the seeing and touching taboos.

While this therapy was first used to help those with considerable emotional discomfort function effectively, anyone can benefit from it. The emotional "problem" it deals with is body prejudice. Variations of some of the methods and techniques used can be applied to your own life.

Nude therapy originated in the late 1960s when a few psychologists began encouraging nudity in group therapy situations as an aid to bringing out into the open participants' negative body attitudes. Though these attitudes affect the way a person views himself in relationship to other people, they frequently do not surface in conventional therapy. Paul Bindrim, a clinical psychologist in Los Angeles, was one of the first to develop specific techniques involving the use of nudity in a therapy situation.

Bindrim's first experience came about quite by accident and not because of any interest in nudity per se. He discovered that his therapy groups seemed to make quicker progress when they camped out and did their work in beautiful outdoor surroundings. During one of these camping trips he saw how being nude with others could bring about therapeutic results. The insight came because his therapy group wanted to visit the hot baths at Esalen Growth Center, near their Big Sur campgrounds. When the group arrived at Esalen they found, to their surprise, people of both sexes bathing naked together. The group decided to join them. Bindrim recalls:

> There was one very shy man in the group—about 55, I guess. And scared to death of sex, women, and dating. He was a real candidate for early senility. That night he sat naked in the tubs with the others and splashed and frolicked like a baby, saying excitedly, "It's me. My God, it's me." Following that experience he made some remarkable breakthroughs in his individual therapy sessions with me. Within a year, he was having normal sexual relations. I saw something very profound happening there—something I never would have predicted. It was all background material and you need a lot of

background material before you can try anything new. But it got me thinking that nudity could be of use in the therapeutic process.

At about the time of Bindrim's experience Dr. Abraham Maslow (then President of the American Psychological Association and considered the father of the human-potential movement) put his seal of approval on the idea that nudity could be a useful therapeutic tool. In his 1965 book, *Eupsychian Management*, he said that "going naked before a lot of other people, is itself a kind of therapy, especially if we can be conscious of it, that is, if there's a skilled person around to direct what's going on, to bring things to consciousness."

Bindrim had been accustomed to organizing psychological "marathons," a therapeutic technique in which participants meet in continuous session from eighteen to forty-eight hours in order to mutually explore and enhance their emotional growth under the guidance of a leader. When he became convinced of the therapeutic benefits of nudity, Bindrim joined with sociologists William Hartman and Marilyn Fithian of California State University, Long Beach, to organize a nude marathon. Held one weekend in June, 1967, at Deer Park, a nudist camp in California, the marathon, probably the first of its kind, was limited primarily to psychologists, psychiatrists, marriage counselors, and others with considerable experience in conventional group and individual therapy. Even so, it (and subsequent nude marathons) drew considerable comment from the mass media and even the psychological community. Bindrim was harassed by phone calls and outraged letters. The Ethics Committee of the American Psychological Association investigated him to determine if he had violated any of the codes of the profession. Apparently he hadn't since the inquiry was terminated without any action being taken.

Today nude therapy is a recognized, if not widely accepted, technique. Papers on the subject have been presented at many universities and at the conventions of both the American Psychological Association, the Association of Humanistic Psychology, and the American Psychiatric Association. Nudity has become a useful therapeutic tool, especially for body and sex therapists.

NUDE MARATHONS CAN LEAD TO
BODY ACCEPTANCE—AND SELF-ACCEPTANCE

The previously mentioned nude marathon was made up of twelve men and twelve women, from college age to the fifties. On a Friday night after a discussion on why nudity was being introduced as part of the therapeutic process, the group members undressed and gathered close together in a warm whirlpool bath. Later in the evening color slides projected on their bodies as they danced and swayed and posed.

In the morning the group members awoke relaxed and alert—and amazed that the nudity and touching hadn't led to sex. They took a nature hike through the park, maintaining silence to let new insights and thoughts fall into place. The rest of Saturday and all day Sunday was devoted to the activities usually undertaken at conventional therapy weekends. The intensity of the therapy occasionally was relieved by jacuzzi breaks—play gatherings in the swirling 100° plus water where the tensions of therapy were dissipated in laughing, joking, and joyous non-sexual body contact.

The weekend ended with a "peak experience" technique for bringing deep and tender emotions to awareness. Each participant listened to a favorite musical recording, held in his hand something he had brought with him that was pleasing to touch (a smooth rock, a piece of soft or silky material, etc.), smelled something he enjoyed (lemon blossoms, perfume, spices, etc.), tasted something he found particularly delicious, and focused on a significant experience in his life that had given him pleasure.

In evaluating the weekend most participants concluded that removing the "mask" of clothing had helped in breaking down the barriers that keep people from feeling close to one another and being honest with each other. Many reported having what might be called a spiritual experience —the feeling of being truly in harmony with nature and other people.

Pleasurable experiences were not the only results. Studies have supported what the participants of this early nude marathon believed to be true—nude therapy can have long-lasting and beneficial effects. For example, in 1974, for his doctoral dissertation at the California School of Professional Psychology, Paul Wheatley compared the effects of nude and clothed marathons, concluding the nude groups resulted in more positive changes—the changes still apparent six months after the marathon.

Some of the ways in which participants changed were as follows:

They learned to like themselves better.
They showed an increased desire for relationships with others.
They experienced an increased ability to make contact with others.
They demonstrated an increased ability to live in the present and make effective use of their time.

Nudity Can Be Therapeutic

Many of the positive changes brought about in Bindrim's groups—particularly the greater self-acceptance and better relationships with others—are also some of the positive changes that can come about through body liberation. In fact, Emily (and the many therapists and group leaders who now utilize nudity as a therapeutic tool) use many of Bindrim's techniques including a pool of warm water and carefully structured, safe (non-sexual) body contact.

Encouraging the removal of clothing in group therapy is based on a belief that the exposure of a person's body to others can help him discover his feelings about his appearance. In addition, the removal of symbolic defenses—clothing—can help break down psychological defenses and help a person learn to interact more openly and honestly with others. Because we believe in the benefits of nudity, we have included in this book many suggestions on how you can use your own nude body as your major learning aid in the process of liberating your body.

Probably the most important aspect of Bindrim's nude therapy is that it allows body contact without sex. An experience such as this helps dispel the erroneous belief that keeps people from getting their much needed rations of touching—the belief that touching, particularly touching with tenderness, will inevitably lead to sex.

Many people suffer from "skin-to-skin hunger," a hunger satisfied by controlled skin contact. Such contact can lead to what Bindrim considers a spiritual experience:

Spiritual, if it means anything, means returning to the source. And when you take off the markings of your differentness, when you remove your clothing, when you're in the water, so many things that separate us disappear—particularly when touch is permitted. When nonsexually oriented touch is permitted in the water, even the sense of male and femaleness is lost. People are people. Age disappears. Professional status disappears. It is a returning to the source. And when bodies are floated, stroked, and slowly passed between two rows of people and there is beautiful music playing, it's like watching human beings being born, as though they came out of the great source of all life and poured out across the pool. People have expressed how wonderful it is to feel that they are simply a part of this whole life process and to feel that union again. That union, that sense of sameness, is the essence of the spiritual experience.

Scientists are beginning to verify what pioneers such as Bindrim have observed—touch is a form of nourishment humans need in their daily diets as much as they need the food they eat. We need touching, plenty of it every day. We need lots of hugs, strokes, and pats in order to be emotionally healthy, loving and lovable, efficient and productive.

The idea that *satisfying body contact is a basic human need that must be fulfilled* (not only for positive good health but for normal physical and emotional development) is developed by anthropologist Ashley Montagu in his book, *Touching: The Human Significance of the Skin*... "to a very significant extent, a measure of the individual's development as a healthy human being is the extent to which he or she is freely able to embrace another and enjoy the embraces of others—to get, in a very real sense, into touch with others."

According to Montagu, the adult who is not "in touch" with others (usually because of childhood tactile deprivation) tends to be clumsy not only in his physical relations with others (kissing, hugging, shaking hands, sex), but in his verbal exchanges. Frequently such a person lacks tact and is socially inept. Touching, says Montagu, serves to "give the individual the reassurance that he needs, the conviction that he is wanted and valued, and thus involved and consolidated in a connected network of values with others."

Nude groups provide touch-starved adults with an opportunity to receive loving, nonsexual body contact.

BABIES NEED TOUCHING

If touch is important to adults, it is vital to babies for their normal development—sometimes for their very survival. (In a later chapter, we'll tell you how to incorporate the principles of body liberation into your family life.) Here are some findings on the importance of touch.

Babies can die from a lack of body contact. In the early part of this century, many babies in foundling homes and hospitals used to die of a mysterious "wasting-away" disease called *marasmus*. The disease was cured only when doctors—suspecting the link between lack of sufficient mothering and marasmus—began prescribing tender, loving care. Nurses and attendants picked up the babies at regular intervals and hugged, fondled, rocked, stroked, and cuddled them. The mortality rate at the homes dropped dramatically.

There is evidence that loving skin stimulation can also be helpful to an infant's neurological development. Premature infants—kept in incubators at the hospital and handled gingerly and infrequently by nervous parents when they go home—often suffer physical and mental disabilities.

In an effort to discover if any of these disabilities resulted not from the prematurity, but from the lack of touching, Dallas psychologist Ruth Rice trained fifteen mothers of premature infants in stroking, rocking, and massaging treatments designed to stimulate nerve pathways. When the babies were released from the hospital, the mothers began the treatments. The infants who had received this body contact from their mothers demonstrated, upon being tested at the age of four months, greater weight gains, higher scores in mental functioning, and greater neurological development than the premature babies who hadn't had this body contact.

Children who are touch-deprived may develop a variety of emotional and physiological problems—including a tendency toward violence. This thesis is supported by psychologist James W. Prescott of the National Institute of Child Health and Human Development.

Prescott based his conclusions on two main sources. The first were laboratory studies by Harry F. and Margaret K. Harlow at the University of Wisconsin, who found that monkeys reared alone in cages (though still able to see, hear, and smell other monkeys) all exhibited abnormal behaviors such as rocking and head banging—behaviors identical to those developed by some touch-deprived children in institutions. The second source was Prescott's study of child-rearing practices, sexual behavior, and violence in forty-nine primitive societies. He found that in societies where much physical affection was permitted or encouraged, there was less physical violence than in societies where body contact was discouraged.

Prescott's evidence would seem to suggest that some of our present social problems might be attributed to lack of touching as much as to poverty or moral decay or television, other frequently cited causes. Prescott says in *The Futurist* magazine: "the deprivation of body touch, contact, and movement are the basic causes of a number of emotional disturbances which include depressive and autistic behaviors, hyperactivity, sexual aberration, drug abuse, violence, and aggression."

Because of studies such as these and the proven effectiveness of touch in helping people who are troubled emotionally, the health professions are beginning to discover what healers have known since the beginning of man—the laying-on-of-hands can be an effective therapeutic technique. More and more people in the health professions are acknowledging the importance of touch to good health. Nurses are encouraged to take courses in therapeutic touch and psychotherapists are learning how to combine touch with words to facilitate the healing of emotional pains. Even ancient stress-relieving touches such as acupressure (applying pressure to certain points in the body) are being rediscovered.

The discovery of the body's need for touch holds as much promise for well-being as did the earlier discovery of the body's need for vitamins. This discovery, as with vitamins, is creating new professions and practices that contribute to better health and more enjoyment.

One such new therapeutic system was developed by Dr. John F. Thie. It utilizes acupressure, touch, and massage to improve postural balance and reduce physical and mental pain and tension. In his book *Touch for Health* (written with Mary Marks), Dr. Thie says it is important that we learn to touch each other for reasons other than sex or punishment (our two most common reasons for making physical contact with another person's body). He explains, "Even with children, touching is looked upon with suspicion. But now we have another reason to touch—to help each other. We can touch for health."

French physician Frederick Leboyer has made the infant's need for touch the basis for a new theory of obstetrics, which he calls "birth without violence." The attending physician at a Leboyer type of delivery tries to make the baby's transition from womb to outside world less traumatic—to show him that this new place is going to be okay. The doctor handles the baby slowly and carefully—stroking and gently massaging him. The baby is not separated from his mother immediately but lies on her chest enjoying the warmth and closeness and hearing her familiar heartbeat. To ease the shock of adjusting to a strange new world, the infant is also immersed for a time in warm water—a wet and soothing environment similar to the one he just left. It's no wonder that brand new Leboyer babies have a relaxed, rather than a tortured, countenance and that some of them even smile.

Compare the Leboyer method with what happens to babies delivered in the conventional way. Babies are greeted on their entrance into their new environment not with loving touch but with a series of rude shocks; they are held upside down and slapped, they hear a lot of noise and see harsh, glaring lights, they are separated almost immediately from the person to whom they have been intimately joined for nine months.

When the infant goes home—even to the most loving parents—he will probably not be cuddled and caressed and rocked and hugged as much as he should be. Ashley Montagu criticizes the impersonal child-rearing practices in this country which put barriers—blankets, caps, booties, nightgowns, bottles, cribs, etc.—between an infant and his parents. A baby first perceives the world he is going to live in through his sense of touch and his earliest (and most important) perceptions are likely to be of material things—not warm, living human skin. If a baby's groping hands always encounter a button instead of a warm chest, a sweater instead of an arm, or rough fabric instead of a soft tummy, perhaps his world is apt to seem somewhat impersonal and materialistic. Since a baby's first impressions lay the foundation for the way he will view life, such treatment is bound to inhibit his behavior and restrict his pleasure as an adult.

ADULTS NEED TOUCHING

As adults we restrict both the number of people it is okay to touch and the occasions when it is okay to touch them. For example, babies, young children, sexual partners, and animals may be caressed, cuddled, held, hugged, stroked or petted. Almost everyone else is off limits except in superficial ways. Men can shake hands and slap each other on the back. Women can give each other a peck on the cheek when saying hello or good-bye. We can kiss the bride at weddings and embrace the bereaved at funerals. But much of the time our bodies are not touched in any way at all by other bodies, or if they are, we feel uneasy. If you are sitting next to a friend and accidentally touch him with your arm or body, you are more likely to excuse yourself and quickly move away than to relax and enjoy the contact. If someone of the opposite sex wants to rub your back, you probably suspect the gesture to be a sexual overture. A woman recently wrote a poignant, and all too typical, letter to one of the advice columnists in the newspapers complaining that her husband rarely touched her but that the first thing he did when he got home from work was to hug, pet, scratch, fondle, and romp with—his dog.

Because of social taboos against touching, it is usual for adults to touch one another in but three ways—ritualistically (e.g., shaking hands), during sex, and when fighting. Meaningless bed-hopping may be the result of an unconscious desire for more touching; one reason dangerous body-contact sports are so popular may be because of the need for a socially acceptable way to prevent touch-starvation. There are better ways, and one purpose of this book is to introduce some of them and hasten their acceptance.

There is a whole range of enjoyable ways to touch and be touched. Some of these ways can be discovered within the safe framework of professionally led groups that permit certain kinds of touching but which do not permit violence or sexual activity. In a nude therapy group or at a workshop led by a skilled group leader the rules of the outside world can be temporarily suspended. In a controlled and supervised setting participants can give and receive what they have been consciously or unconsciously craving in their everyday lives—the loving touch of other human beings.

Another way to get your fair share of touching is to practice with a partner some of the exercises suggested later in this book. Who knows, maybe someday the government will develop a minimal-daily-requirement list for touching.

If the thought of joining a group, taking a class, or trying some new techniques to improve your ability to touch and be touched doesn't appeal to you, we are not surprised. You've been living within the confines of our society's body taboos. As a result you may feel no need for more touching; you may feel you are touched more than you would like to be.

We understand. Not too long ago, had anyone tried to talk with us about nudity or touching, especially had they tried to convince us that either could enrich our lives, we would have backed away in a hurry. We would have considered such ideas bizarre. But somewhere along the line we began to realize that although it appeared we were content, something important was missing from our lives. Slowly and cautiously, we began opening doors and widening our horizons. This expansion of our lives brought us in contact with almost every experience, place, and idea that is in this book. In the process of breaking through the seeing and touching taboos of our society, we discovered a whole new dimension to life. We hope we can entice you into some cautious explorations that will do the same for you.

Chapter 6
Being Born Again

> Seeing, hearing, feeling, are miracles, and each part and tag of me is a miracle.
>
> Walt Whitman,
> *Song of Myself*

At middle-age, we, the authors, experienced a rebirth that profoundly changed us and our worlds. Our "midwives" were the loving and accepting people we met as we searched—on our own, in groups, with friends and professionals in many fields—for the missing elements in our lives and in ourselves. These people not only provided us with exciting new insights and ideas, but they also looked at our bodies, touched and accepted them—and us—just as we are.

Our rebirth was sometimes painful, but out of the pain came a greater sense of self-acceptance, improved relationships, and a whole new way of life. In reentering the world in a new way, we had begun the process of liberating our bodies. Because we know how hard it is to achieve and maintain a liberated body in a body prejudiced world, we decided to write this book. We want to help others have a second birth, a gentle "Leboyer" birth, and we want to help bring about the kind of world where a liberated body will be a birthright for all.

EMILY'S STORY

If you were to pick from a crowd the person least likely to write a book about nudity, it would be me. I look like what I am—a middle-aged, middle-class lady. Most of my adult life has been devoted not to bodies and nudity but to my family and to a career running a medical laboratory with my husband. During my twenty-nine year marriage I managed our large home in Long Beach, California, and raised two sons. As our business prospered, I also learned to manage our stock portfolio and the two apartment houses we were eventually able to buy. I was busy and I thought I was content.

But in 1963 I was selected by the adult-education department of UCLA as one of sixty-eight women in Southern California to participate in an experimental seminar to develop the personal and social potential of women. That seminar changed the direction of my life. I realized I had never taken time to look inside myself to find out what I really wanted to do and what I was really capable of doing.

The seminar led me to search for self-discovery through the study of a wide range of subjects—humanistic psychology, sociology, cultural anthropology, existential philosophy, Oriental religions, communication techniques, creative writing, and more. Encounter groups and workshops gave me further insight into my own desires and potential. I learned that what I really wanted to do was motivate others to shake up their lives in pleasurable ways, to find the joy that I was finding. I found I had the ability to help others with their personal growth and began giving workshops aimed at increasing self-esteem and improving interpersonal relationships.

As I learned more about myself and how I wanted to live in my second half-century, my husband and I discovered we no longer had similar goals, no longer wanted the same lifestyle. Because we cared deeply for each other and did not want to stand in the way of one another's happiness, we decided to part.

My life changed rapidly. Hoping to adjust to a new unmarried state I attended a weekend workshop for singles held at Elysium Field in Topanga, a growth center where the wearing of clothing is optional. There was no disrobing during the workshop, however, as it had been arranged by an organization that did not permit it. Ed Lange, the founder of Elysium, was also a participant in the workshop. He sensed the uneasy feelings I had about my body, and when the workshop concluded at noon on Sunday he invited me to stay through the afternoon and meet some people who might be able to teach me something about how to become comfortable with my body. Ed assured me I would be under no pressure to take off my clothes. Being at a painful stage in my life I knew I had to do some things that might be frightening because they were unfamiliar—and "naked" was as unfamiliar as "single"—so I stayed.

Sitting in my bathing suit beside the pool that Sunday afternoon, I watched as the regular members of Elysium arrived, bringing children, picnic baskets, and beach balls. After spreading out towels and blankets, they shed their clothes, and most of them headed for the pool.

It was a hot August day. Playing in the pool was the most logical thing to do. However, since everyone else was naked, I was afraid my going in the water wearing a suit would seem odd. With much trepidation, I took off my suit and slipped into the water. There was no bolt of lightning from the sky.

The water was refreshing, the people were friendly—the sensation of freedom and release I felt was exhilarating.

Then parts of bodies touched mine. The pool was almost overflowing with people—moving people, naked people. I kept swimming, trying to avoid people until I was exhausted.

Yet, though uncomfortable at being touched, I realized I also liked it. I needed to sit and sort out my thoughts and feelings.

I looked around for a place to climb out of the pool where no one would see me. There was no such place. The pool was rimmed with naked people stretched out, sunning themselves.

Slowly I made my way to the shallow end of the pool figuring that if I fainted before I got out because people were looking at me, at least I wouldn't drown. As I got out, the worst possible thing happened. I saw a man I had known for years.

"Emily," he said, passing by, "I never realized what a good body you have."

He meant it so obviously as a genuine compliment and not as a sexual overture that my embarrassment and fear vanished.

However, I also realized that I saw naked women as individuals but naked men as shapeless, gray, nebulous, unknowable creatures. It occurred to me that I had always related to men and women in these terms. I also started thinking about how I confused nudity and sex, frequently associating an honest compliment about my body with a sexual pass. I had always tried to avoid compliments about my body. I had not gone naked in our home or in the one I grew up in. In the Catholic convent school I attended as a child I was taught that bodies should be covered at all times and that it was unthinkable to be in the bathroom with somebody else. Getting married didn't change my feelings about my body, especially its sexual parts. The man I married was also uptight about anyone seeing his body. Our sons soon picked up our taboos. When they were about ten, both decided no one was ever going to see them unclothed or even in their underwear.

I Learn to Accept Myself Unclothed

These thoughts made me want to try something daring and scary—walk around the Elysium grounds naked, no makeup on, hair wet and streaming. Several people looked at me and spoke to me, treating me easily and respectfully. They accepted me in my most exposed state. And I found I was able to accept myself unclothed. I felt wonderful.

After the Elysium experience I began to feel other releasing kinds of changes taking place in me. For instance, for the first time in my life I was able to stand up and speak before a large audience. I realized the reason for my previous difficulty was the fear of being seen as I really was, without a facade, and of being found inadequate. I no longer felt that way. I also began designing special programs to help unmarried people improve their relationships with members of the opposite sex and live fuller lives; programs with titles such as "How To Be Happily *Un*married," "Making Friends with the Opposite Sex," and "Touch and Go: Short-Term Relationships." I conducted them for universities, churches, singles clubs, and growth centers throughout the United States and in Canada, Mexico, England, Spain, and Tahiti.

I wanted to help other people—other nice, proper people like me—learn how to come to terms with their own bare bodies. Since most adults consider a suggestion to take off their clothes as tantamount to proposing an orgy, I decided to design workshops that would make disrobing and talking about bodies safe, easy, fun, and educational. A good place to conduct the workshops seemed to be at Elysium Field.

Elysium was being developed into an unusual kind of human-potential center, where people could learn to rid themselves of body taboos and the neurotic behavior accompanying these taboos. I was offered a job as its first program director.

As I began to compare the progress made by those in Elysium's "clothing optional" environment with that made in my more conventional workshops (at universities and other institutions), I had to conclude that those attending Elysium learned more quickly. They also became friendly more quickly in nude groups. They listened more attentively to one another, were more cooperative, and there was more laughter and fun. Nudity seemed to be an educational device that could be used effectively in many, many ways.

While nude camps, nude beaches, and nude therapy had laid the groundwork, nudity in educational environments seemed needed for more effective teaching of body health, knowledge, and stress-free pleasure.

I Begin to Use Nudity as a Liberating Tool

I began to look for new ways to use nudity as an educational tool, ways that would offer more people opportunities to learn about body prejudice and how to rid themselves of it. To reach more people than those who went to Elysium I designed a short, body-image-improvement workshop that could be given anywhere that three hours of privacy were assured. (Called "Brave Nude World," it is described in a later chapter.) I also began designing programs emphasizing "holistic nudity"—programs that stress the integration of body and mind, helping people to appreciate the complexity, beauty, and wonder of their bodies, to take care of their bodies in new and better ways, to show them off more often, and to enjoy them more thoroughly. I gave numerous day-long, weekend, and weekly clothing-optional workshops, with such titles as "Developing Your Personal Potential," "Enhancing Your Sex Life," "Dare to Be Daring," "Learn to Talk and Be

Heard," etc. For a couple of years, I also conducted "Sunday Services" in the nude—a two-hour Sunday afternoon program free to anyone who visited Elysium. It was designed to inspire people to feel good about themselves, other people, and the world.

Many of the concepts and techniques I developed during the eight years I conducted programs on "holistic nudity" are included in this book. I am convinced that no matter what activity is taking place—a workshop, seminar, meeting, party, or family gathering—when people are able to look at and talk about their bodies, touch one another with affection, express their feelings and their thoughts, more mutual understanding and learning will take place.

By 1972, I had written a book, *Making Friends with the Opposite Sex* (Nash Publishing Co.) which was well-received. I wanted to write another to share my knowledge of the benefits of body liberation with people who might never come to a place like Elysium or participate in a clothing-optional workshop. However, I had found writing to be a lonely process, and wanted a partner to work with me on this book, a partner who had a background that would complement mine but who also would add new dimensions and viewpoints. I also wanted someone who possessed a considerable amount of self-awareness so that we could resolve the inevitable problems and pressures of working closely with another person. Finally, I wanted someone who would be fun to be around, for I had learned that I could do my best work only when I felt good and enjoyed myself while working. I found this special partner when Betty Edwards, a participant in one of my clothing-optional singles workshops at Elysium, introduced herself as a writer and asked to interview me. That interview resulted in a friendship, a creative collaboration, and ultimately this book.

BETTY'S STORY

Like Emily, I, too, would seem to be an unlikely person to write a book on body liberation. At the time I agreed to collaborate, I did not consider myself an expert on nudity and definitely did not *want* to be considered one.

At one time I had wanted recognition in the academic world, an achievement that did not come easily since I didn't start my full-time college education until after the birth of my third child. However, eventually I earned a master's degree in history, acquiring in the process a background in political science, cultural anthropology, and cultural and political geography. I began teaching high school in 1963 where I gained some reputation as an innovator for devising techniques and games to make history more palatable to the students and for making the classroom a place where students felt free to express themselves. When my marriage of twenty-four years ended, I added another dimension to my professional life, that of free-lance writer. I wrote magazine and newspaper articles on such subjects as education, politics, and the environment, urging people to think about the serious social problems we all face.

My ambition was to write a book that would help make the world a better place. Writing a book about bodies not only would have struck me as a waste of time but also would have seemed to be a threat to my reputation and my self-respect. The development of this book demonstrated I had not even had my self-respect to lose. I had not had body pride.

By the time I met Emily I had become more receptive to new ideas. I had already tried disrobing with others, once somewhat incidentally in the baths at Esalen, during an intensive week-long Gestalt workshop, another time during one of Emily's singles workshops at Elysium. Although I was impressed with Emily and her leadership abilities, going bare to me was still sort of an adventure—the kind of activity that would allow me to brag of my daring. But I certainly didn't consider nudity an important subject.

I Try Clothing My Nudity in Detachment

Whatever my original reservations, I had a writer's sense of commitment, and as Emily and I threw ourselves into the book I spent a great deal of time reading, researching, and interviewing. We would not ask our readers to try anything we had not done ourselves, and since Emily viewed going bare as being so natural, it was up to me to experience what it felt like for a newcomer to social nudity.

I visited nude resorts, beaches, and workshops, and engaged in techniques and games I wouldn't have tried without the impetus of the book. I even invented some. A lot of emotion resulted from these activities, but in the early stages I handled it by maintaining the detachment of a researcher or reporter. After all, I wasn't really into this stuff; I was just helping to write a book about it. But detachment could not last.

One weekend at the beginning of our research, Emily and I had gone to interview the owner of a nude trailer-camp and his clientele. During the day I talked to people, swam, and hiked, all in the nude, and congratulated myself on being able to be so open to this new experience. That night, however, we were invited to stay over in order to avoid a long drive home after dark, and I found that nudity at night inside the trailer produced quite different feelings than it did during the day. Though Emily and the owner were casually and comfortably unclothed, I was reluctant to remove the robe I had donned in the late afternoon for warmth. Outdoor daytime nudity seemed natural and appropriate; indoor nighttime nudity—in close quarters with a person of the opposite sex—had too many sexual connotations. Although I knew our host expected no sex from us, I feared he might "lose control" and try to "get us into an orgy."

Unable to express these feelings, I announced I was tired, and with my robe still on, climbed into my sleeping bag. Then, all the while making a pretense of chatting casually with the other two, I wriggled out of my robe under the covers. Emily barely kept a straight face as I frantically maneuvered to prevent my host from catching a tiny glimpse of what he had been viewing all day long.

In the morning Emily and I talked about my fears, and I realized I was simply being an *external* nudist—one who allows his body to receive the health and pleasure benefits of nudity but who is not truly comfortable with his body or sexuality. It was through many discussions like these (sometimes with much tears and laughter) that Emily and I evolved many of the suggestions in this book. My reactions to nudity gave Emily new insights; she helped me sort out my emotions.

At the time I was abandoning my detached attitude toward work on the book I had a dream in which I was back in my role of wife and my husband and I were visiting friends. In the bizarre way that dreams operate I suddenly needed to change my clothes and started undressing in front of everyone. My husband and friends looked at me with such horror that I quickly covered myself.

"But," I said, "you knew I was writing a book on nudity, and you thought it was okay."

"Writing about it is one thing," they answered coldly. "Doing it is another."

From that point on the book became a personal commitment. I realized I had been worried that writing the book would make me unacceptable socially and professionally, and that I was saying body liberation was okay for readers but not for me. Once I made the commitment I began accepting all of me—not just my mind and intellect but also my less-than-physically-perfect body. And I found that others accepted my body, too. I also learned to accept my sexuality, my physical functions, my womanliness. My female anatomy became natural and wholesome to me, a source of aesthetic pleasure rather than shame.

Accepting My Body Increased My Self-Esteem

I am a different person now from when we started working on this book. I feel better about myself and that feeling shows. It shows in the care I take of my body and in my increased self-esteem. It shows in the deeper and more loving relationships I have with my family and friends. I learned that I could comfortably and unashamedly go bare with male and female friends—massaging each other and sharing feelings about our bodies. I also learned to admit I needed other human beings.

In addition, I am regaining an ability I once had to take pleasure in the most inexpensive and easily available resource around—my own body. Often when I least expect it—when soaking in a jacuzzi, dancing to rock music, walking on the beach, hugging a friend—I experience a sense of sheer, indescribable physical pleasure. My body becomes light, free, joyous. I am experiencing body joy.

Chapter 7
Realizing Body Joy

> I live in my body like a spirit in a cloud.
>
> Isadora Duncan, *My Life*

Everyone has known body joy. We knew it as children when we ran up the stairs two at a time just for the sheer pleasure of running, when we skipped instead of walked, when we slid down a bannister or rolled down a grassy hillside in sheer abandon, letting our bodies go where they wanted to go and stop when they wanted to stop. Though most grownups reared in a body prejudiced society have lost much of their inborn ability to experience body joy, there are some exceptions. Every day of their lives, some people experience pleasure through full use of their senses. Isadora Duncan was such a person.

In the early part of this century she helped liberate dance as an art form. She tossed aside costumes that restricted movement as well as the rigid and stylized dance patterns typical of the times. Clad in a filmy, flowing tunic, she had a sense of body joy as she moved that captivated audiences in this country and Europe. Neither the loss of her youth nor her figure diminished her sensory pleasure or her appeal. When she wrote the words at the beginning of this chapter, she was in her forties and overweight; yet people flocked to see her perform, absorbing her joyousness.

All of us have the opportunity to reawaken our senses, to recapture much of our childhood abilities to enjoy our bodies. Robert Rimmer, in *The Humanist*,* captures the essence of body joy:

---

*This article, "Flying Naked with my Granddaughter " first appeared in *The Humanist*, November/December 1975, and is reprinted with permission.

"It was early evening—a warm summer night. Followed by her father and mother, our two-and-a-half-year-old granddaughter burst into our house. 'Grampy Bob,' she yelled, shedding her shoes and her tiny print dress and panties. 'Come fly with me.'

"Grandfathers living in middle-class suburbias aren't supposed to teach their grandchildren the joy of being a naked bird. But having raised two sons in 'an environment of being naked when it's convenient to be naked,' it isn't difficult to continue the tradition to a third generation. In a few seconds, I too am naked. Singing a song.... I flap my arms and fly around the yard behind Melissa, admiring her tight buttocks and enjoying a fleeting image of the woman she will become.

"A fifty-six-year generation gap ceases to exist. I revert to my childhood. For a few delightful moments I experience altered consciousness. I regain a childhood ability to both see and live in another reality."

We are going to give you some practically foolproof "recipes" that will help you create body joy for yourself. Some recipes are our own favorites; others come from colleagues in the field of body liberation. Not only do we hope that you will try some or all of them (none are either illegal, immoral, or fattening), but we also hope these will stimulate you to create some of your own recipes. It is our dream that people will someday exchange suggestions for things to do to please the body as freely as they now exchange recipes for concoctions to please the palate.

Most of our recipes don't involve many ingredients. All you need is your own body and a few simple things found around your house or yard. While these experiences can be enjoyed with or without clothes, additional benefits come with nudity. Nudity allows the living fabric that covers you, your skin, to fully experience your environment—the warming rays of the sun on a day in early spring, the play of a gentle breeze all over the body, the tingling coolness of a swim, the sensuous pleasure of a hot springs, feeling languorous on a sultry summer afternoon.

While pleasure alone should be reason enough for nudity, there are health benefits as well. Skin is an extremely important sense organ. Making up 16 to 18 percent of our total body weight, it is loaded with receptors (about 50 per 100 square millimeters of skin) to let us know when we feel cold or heat or pain or other stimuli on our bodies. However, habitually covering our skin with clothing has diminished our skin's ability to respond to stimulation. Just as we would not want to cut down on our ability to see by continually wearing dark glasses when inside the house, it makes no sense to "blind" our skin by always covering-up our bodies. Thus the body joy recipes we have selected emphasize opening the "eyes" of your skin.

Because tactile stimulation from your own hands is a readily available source of body joy, we suggest you begin with a self-massage designed for this book by William Mueller and some of his students at Mueller College of Massage (San Diego, California).

BODY JOY RECIPE 1:
SELF-MASSAGE

Give yourself plenty of time and make sure you won't be interrupted. Supplies you need are towels and oil—baby oil, coconut oil, vegetable oil, or our "loving massage" oil (made by mixing two parts vegetable oil, one part mineral oil, and a few drops of oil of cloves).

1. Run the water in the tub. Have the water as warm as you can comfortably tolerate (remember you will be in the tub awhile and the water will cool).
2. While the water is running, stand in front of a full-length mirror and liberally oil yourself all over.
3. Get in the tub and massage each part of your body in turn using these suggested strokes:

Toes: Massage toes in circular motions; bend, pull, and feel them.

Foot: Arch—rub with thumbs and knuckles; Ball—use thumbs; Heel—squeeze. Grip foot with both hands, one on each side with thumbs in the middle. Pull thumbs to either side to spread bottom of foot in a line from below the toes to the heel. Do this a number of times. Use pumice stone on callouses.

Ankle: Using both hands, move the skin over the underlying tissues. Adjust pressure as desired. Then while holding ankle with one hand, rotate the foot with the other.

Calf: Use stroking movement up and down, knead calf with thumbs. Move skin over muscles with hands. Roll the muscle around the leg bone. Beat gently with fists.

Knee: Move skin around over knee bone using the fingers. Wiggle kneecap.

Abdomen and Chest: Stroke up and down. Cross back and forth (left to right and right to left with both hands). Clockwise movement over abdomen. *Women*: Massage breasts with circular movements clockwise and counterclockwise.

Shoulders: Stroke shoulder, knead, and then stroke again.

Neck: Stroke neck with both hands, pulling down from base of skull.

Head: Move skin behind the ears with fingers, using small circular movement. Work upward above the ears, massaging the scalp with the same small circular movements. Do forehead the same way.

Face: Stroke upward on the face. Move skin over the underlying tissues with small circular movements. Tap face with fingers. Slap face gently.

Arms: Begin with fingers stroking toward the heart. Knead palm of hand with thumb (of opposite hand). Stroke back of hand towards heart. Stroke the arm with upward movement. Move skin over underlying tissues with a twisting movement. Slap arms. Then stroke towards heart.

4. Imagine your eyes are in your fingers, and move your fingers very lightly over your entire body, feeling the texture of the skin, the muscles under the skin, and the bones in your body.

5. Place a hot cloth over your face and relax.

6. Use a shower to soap down and rinse off. Shampoo your hair—and brush your teeth (imagine standing under a waterfall or in the rain in the mountains).

7. Dry off. Put cologne, body lotion, powder, or body oil on yourself.

8. Stand in front of a fan and feel the air blowing over your body.

9. Stretch out for a nap.

BODY JOY RECIPE 2: CHILDLIKE PLAY

You don't have to be a child to experience childlike pleasures. You can encourage the expressive, responsive, sensual child in you to come out and play. Childlike play is much less expensive than a vacation to a faraway resort, or liquor, or tranquilizers. Both indoors and outdoors you can find many toys to play with—some provided by nature and some that are part of the ordinary equipment of your home. With or without clothes, you will find that these activities bring out the child you once were and the body joy you once felt.

Outdoors:

Next time it rains, run around or dance in the rain.
Turn on the sprinklers and run through the water.
Swing in your child's swing or climb on his jungle gym.
Climb a tree.
Roll in the grass.
Take a sun bath.
Take a wind bath.
Pour a bucket of water over your body or hold the hose so that the water goes straight up and then stand underneath it.
Play in the mud. Take the hose and make yourself a good-sized mud puddle—one big enough to sit in. Squish mud between your toes. Cover your body with great handfuls of it. Caution: watch out for sticks, stones, or gravel which can hurt or irritate your skin. Don't worry about bugs or worms—they won't hurt you. Play with them.

Skip or hop around your yard.
Hang a hammock in your yard and swing in it.

Indoors:

Roll around on the rug.
Experiment with the feel against your skin of many materials—velour, satin, fur, velvet, corduroy, toweling, cotton, and so on. You can wrap yourself in these materials, roll on them, sleep on them, stand on them or sit on them.
On a hot day turn the fan on your body.
On a cold day blow hot air from a hair dryer on various parts of your body.

BODY JOY RECIPE 3:
THE BABY ROLL

Try the baby roll, designed by dance therapist Sally McClure, in a fairly large room with a rug on the floor, or outside on your lawn. In this exercise you literally roll around like a baby, letting your inner momentum take you where it will. To begin, lie down on your side with your knees close to your chest and your arms folded over your chest. Then open your knees and the momentum will pull you over. Travel across the floor by opening and closing your knees to propel you. Let your arms go where they want. In fact, let your entire body do what it wants—rock from side to side, roll completely over, travel across the floor fast or slowly. Tumble, rock, and roll freely, just like a baby. Let yourself make any sounds you want. Become aware of the feelings your bodily movements may evoke.

BODY JOY RECIPE 4:
GETTING IN TOUCH WITH YOUR SURROUNDINGS

This body joy exercise can help open the "eyes" of your skin to new pleasure. Use your entire body to explore a familiar room in an unfamiliar way. Instead of feeling it with your fingers or hands or looking at it with your eyes, you are going to use the sensitive receptors in the surface of your skin all over your body. And because you can expand your ability to experience one sense more fully by temporarily cutting off another, keep your eyes closed during this exercise.

Experience the room in many different ways. Slide across the rug on your bottom, rub your back against the wall, climb on top of and underneath furniture, sit on tables and stand on chairs. Use all parts of your body to get in touch with your surroundings: your face, your elbow, your toes, your knees, your stomach, your breasts, the undersides of your arms—the ways are limited only by your imagination. Become aware of how different objects feel to your body— the texture of material and wallpaper, the smoothness of wood, the jagged roughness of a metal sculpture. Focus on the place where your body is making contact and concentrate on that place. What does it feel like to your body?

BODY JOY RECIPE 5:
A SOLITARY SENSORY FEAST

This body joy exercise allows you to take delight in all of your senses—sight, sound, touch, taste, and smell—by making a solitary feast an occasion for sensory joy. It is important to enjoy this feast alone so that you can concentrate on your own sensory responses.

Find a special "shrine" for your feast; a place you enjoy looking at and being in—perhaps under a tree in your backyard, in a colorful alcove in your bedroom, by a cozy fire. Set up your table with place mats and napkins and dishes that you enjoy using—sturdy pottery, fine bone china, or paper plates.

Arrange the food and dishes in ways that are pleasing to your eye; try to select colors and textures that offer some contrast. Imagine that your plate is a canvas and the food your materials for creating a modern art painting. Notice the different colors and forms and see how your painting changes when you remove some food.

Listen to the sounds of your feast—the crackling of the paper napkin as you unfold it, the splashing of the milk as you pour it into a glass, the sound of celery or crackers as you chew. Enjoy the feel of everything—the pottery mug made warm by the coffee inside, the fragile smoothness of your elegant crystal, the nubby texture of a chocolate chip cookie. Chew your food very slowly and notice how it feels against your teeth and tongue and the insides of your cheek. How does it feel when you swallow? Become aware of smells—the aroma of the wine, the scent of flowers on the table, the potpourri of smells emanating from the food you are eating.

During your feast move very slowly—pretend you are wading through a tub of molasses. Take time to savor—to enjoy. Concentrate your thoughts on the joy your feast is bringing to all of your senses.

BODY JOY RECIPE 6: DANCE NAKED WITH MUSIC*

Go into a room by yourself. Put on your favorite music. Throw off your clothes. And dance.

For one hour, in complete privacy, you are going to be naked—physically, emotionally, and psychologically.

This may seem to you an extraordinary thing to do. I agree that most people do not ordinarily shut themselves into a room and dance naked. Nevertheless, put aside shyness, reserve, convention—and do this recipe. There are sound principles behind it, and good values to be gained from it.

You are going to set your body free of all its limitations and inhibitions, set it free to feel the music, to move with it, to be one with it.

This is not an artistic undertaking, so do not judge yourself. Ignore the mirror, or, if you cannot ignore it, cover it. Do not correct your movements; do not even allow yourself to make a mental image of your movements. Do not compare or evaluate—stop judging.

The goal of this dance is not art. The goal is personal freedom.

---

*Reprinted with the permission of Farrar, Straus, & Giroux, Inc. from *You Are Not the Target*, by Laura Archera Huxley, copyright © 1963 by Laura Huxley.

Whether you are nineteen or ninety, whether you weigh one hundred or three hundred pounds, whether you move with ease or difficulty, whether your joints are supple or stiff—no matter. Dance.

This dance is not for anyone's eyes, not even your own.

You are dancing from within, dancing only your feelings, especially your repressed feelings. You are dancing what you cannot tell your mother or father, your husband, lover or friend, what you cannot tell your minister, priest or psychoanalyst, what you cannot tell yourself.

When you are throwing off your clothes, think and feel that you are throwing off all the ideas, feelings, compulsions, embarrassments, fears, and shames that have been *superimposed* upon you. Some of these ideas and restraints are necessary and useful some of the time, but not all of them, and not all of the time. For this dance, throw off everything that has been superimposed upon your real self.

Be whatever you are.

BE—naked and alone.

With the first article of clothing throw off your social status. You may like your status, you may enjoy your social role—no matter. Throw them off.

With the next article of clothing, throw off the blindly accepted conventions of behavior; they may serve you well enough in public. But now, as you get ready to dance, throw them off.

With the third article of clothing, throw off your personal mask, the image of yourself that you present to others. Whatever it is, whether it is an heroic cover for desperation, whether it hides tenderness with a scowl, anxiety with laughter, loneliness with aloofness, resentment with humility—throw it off.

When you come to the last article of clothing, throw off with it the fear, ignorance, and shame that have been imposed upon you by those who lack understanding and respect for sex and love. Throw off that last bit of clothing and that last restraint before you begin your dance.

If it is loneliness you feel, let all your body feel it. If it is rage or hostility or fear, feel it with every cell. Through your naked dance, you expel all the unwanted, painful feelings.

If these feelings become people and faces and colors, look at them. If they haunt you, dance them away. Dance them out, out, out of you.

For one who is an invalid: You can follow the directions for this recipe, using any part of the body that you can move. If any part of you is not free to move, follow the instructions in your imagination. Give a title to your dance and choose the music. Then close your eyes and dance so completely in your imagination that you actually feel the circulation of your blood quickened and stimulated. When, at the end of your dance, you open your eyes, you will feel how much more alive, how much more under your control, and how much more comfortable your body is than before you did this recipe.

Here is a list of feelings. We experience some of these, perhaps all of them, at one time or another. Make one of these the title of your dance or, better, make your own title. Dance one of these:

I am the center of the world, but nobody recognizes it.
I am afraid, but I don't want anybody to know it.
I am afraid, but I don't want to let myself know it.
I am afraid in my imagination.
I do to others that which has been done to me.
I must keep up with the Joneses!
I hate the one I love.
I want to give, give, give, but I don't know how.
I am hiding behind myself.
I am hiding behind the devilish part of myself.
I am hiding behind the angelic part of myself.
I am just too tired to dance out my tiredness.
I do not *have* to keep up with the Joneses!

Or of these:

fear—loneliness—injustice—love—anger—
sexual desire—desire to take—desire to give—
apathy—desire to console—desire to hurt—
too afraid to move—hostility—uncertainty—
inability to do what I want—inability to express
myself—or—

I want to love; I want to be loved.
I want to love; I want to be loved.

Listen and be open to the freer part of yourself when you choose or make a title for your dance.

If you are going to dance an unwanted feeling, one that you want to expel and be rid of, continue with your dance until you know that this feeling no longer interferes with you, psychologically or physiologically.

If you choose to dance a feeling that is precious to you, one that makes your life richer, that augments and expands you—then dance it. Let it take hold of you and strengthen your whole organism. Nourish this feeling, and let it bloom like a flower. Let the dance and the music be the sun and the water that nourish this good feeling.

Change the pace of your dance with this variation:

At any point of your dance—suddenly *stop!*
Become a frozen statue.

At any moment, in any position, stop and stiffen. Make your whole body stiff, stiffer, still stiffer. Think of each part of your body and make it stiff.

Keep it stiff as long as you possibly can.

Do not breathe. Your body is so stiff that you cannot even breathe.

You have made your body so stiff that there can be no movement—no movement at all.

When you are at the limit of your endurance, when your body is so absolutely stiff and so absolutely crying for oxygen, when it is humanly impossible to hold it any longer—let go!

You will experience an immense relaxation and with it a flood of gratitude for the enormous privilege of breathing.

Do this several times during your dance. Remember, each time you do it, that your entire body must be stiff, unmoving, like one single piece of ice.

If one could guarantee anything at all in the area of human reactions, I would guarantee that this recipe, properly done, will bring you a period of complete bodily relaxation and pleasurable comfort.

To summarize the directions:

Decide the title of your dance.

Choose the music.

In rhythm with the music, throw off your clothes. With each piece of clothing, throw off a restraint, a convention, a mask imposed upon you by others or yourself.

Know what each piece of clothing represents. Name it. Know that you are free of it.

Dance. Let the music and your feeling and your body be one. Dance what you feel. BE what you feel. This is your dance. IF you feel like singing—sing. If you feel like shrieking or chanting or wailing, then shriek or chant or wail. This is your dance—your creation—your liberation.

Note: If you do not have a whole hour to dance, then dance for a few minutes, even dressed. Use this recipe whenever you must do something requiring especially controlled behavior; use it before an official function or a difficult interview. If you are going to a party or out with a date, do this recipe. It will freshen and relax you and improve your looks.

It works—if you work.

Chapter 8
Going Bare
with Children

> Being natural and matter-of-fact about nudity prevents your children from developing an attitude of shame or disgust about the human body. If parents are very secretive about their bodies and go to great lengths to prevent their children from ever seeing a buttock or breast, children will wonder what is so unusual and even alarming about human nudity.
>
> Dr. Lee Salk,
McCall's, June 1976

Babies are born without body prejudice. They do not need instruction on how to achieve body joy. They find all parts of their bodies fascinating; no functions disgust them. Babies like to suck, and although they may sometimes prefer a breast or a bottle, if neither is available, their own fingers, hands, or toes will do. No body parts are off limits for exploration. Babies feel no guilt about touching themselves until guilt is taught. A mother may frown when her baby grabs his penis or she may push away his hands when he touches her breasts. A baby has no shame about being seen in his natural, naked state—shame, too, is taught.

PARENTS TEACH THEIR CHILDREN BODY PREJUDICE OR BODY ACCEPTANCE

Every day, with gestures, words, and disapproving looks many parents teach their children to be prejudiced about their bodies—teach them not to touch themselves or allow others to see certain parts, not to talk about certain functions. In the process parents teach attitudes and habits that stand in the way of good physical health, body and mind integration, needed body contact, and much bodily pleasure. It doesn't take long for our initial body acceptance to disappear. Parents, of course, don't realize the far-reaching effects of their behavior. A snappish "Get out of here—can't you see I'm dressing?" when a child accidentally discovers a parent changing clothes; an embarrassed "Why do you want to know that?" to his questions about one of his body functions; punishment when he playfully throws off his clothes on a hot day—all tell him that bodies, particularly naked bodies, are not acceptable.

The body cover-up that begins in the family is not only harmful to parents and children in ways we pointed out early in this book, it also prohibits a valuable learning experience— the opportunity to discover the beauty in the seasons of the body. Just as we appreciate nature more as we go through each season—spring, summer, winter, fall—we can learn to appreciate the body more as we see it going through its seasons from birth to old age. Such a visual education should be part of the process of living.

For a parent, seeing a child naked now and then and seeing the body changes as a child grows from babyhood to adulthood provides a closeness and an emotional understanding of that child not otherwise attainable. This understanding helps a parent accept the seasons of his child—for example, knowing when a child should no longer be treated like a baby. According to one father whose thirteen-year-old daughter still unself-consciously walks around the house naked: "I can see that my daughter is not my baby anymore. I don't just celebrate her birthdays anymore; I celebrate her growth to womanhood. I know that soon she may begin to cover up her body. I will be denied, when she does, a source of genuine pleasure and contact."

Emily, who had not seen her sons without clothing since they were about ten, had signed up as a participant in a clothing-optional workshop at Elysium. Unknown to her, so had her twenty-seven-year-old son, Michael. Before the workshop she was sitting on the lawn with some friends when to her surprise she heard a cheerful, "Hi, Mom." As Emily tells it, "Looking at his body—so beautiful, so masculine, so grown-up—gave me a different sense of him. I realized he was a man, a responsible person, his own person. I was filled with pleasure and pride in the person I had had a part in creating."

Children also benefit from witnessing the seasons of their parent's bodies. A parent without clothing becomes less of an unchanging, formidable, powerful authoritarian figure and more of a constantly changing, sensitive, vulnerable person—more of a human being. This can be of particular value in improving a child's relationship with the father—who not uncommonly is seen exclusively as an authority-figure. It's possible that one reason many children tend to feel more emotionally distant from their fathers than their mothers is because men cover more of their bodies with clothing. Children have less chance to observe their fathers' bodies and to have any physical contact with them without an intervening layer of clothing.

Why do so many families deny themselves the enjoyment, the emotional closeness, the good health, and the learning that is to be gained from the sight and touch of each other's bodies? The most important factor is probably the parent's fear of what the sight of a nude body (especially the sexual parts) will do to children. This fear was articulated by Sigmund Freud, who developed his theories during the body-denigrating Victorian era. Many of his statements reflect a prejudice against the sexual parts of the human body, particularly the female's sexual parts: "Probably no male human being is spared the fright of castration at the sight of a female genital."

One of the basic assumptions underlying Freudian theory is that male genitals are the most desirable kind to have. Supposedly the fear of losing a penis and "penis envy" are basic and potentially harmful motivating factors in children. When a little boy sees a little girl's genitals, he is supposed to assume that she once had a penis and lost it; he will then worry about losing his. According to Freud, when a little girl sees a little boy's penis, she will conclude that something must be wrong with her—that she was meant to have a penis but that something happened to it or it didn't grow right. Freud assumed that children of both sexes would interpret differences as something terrible, not as a fact of nature.

Another Freudian theory is that young children have a tendency to love the parent of the opposite sex and feel rivalry with the parent of the same sex. A girl may blame her mother for somehow depriving her of a penis and a boy may resent his father's larger penis. Supposedly, if children see their parents nude, it can create anxieties about their own anatomy and intensify the feelings of rivalry for the same-sexed parent and the sexual fantasies about the opposite-sexed parent.

Freudian theory reaches parents because of its influence on such child-rearing authorities as Dr. Benjamin Spock, who discussed his views on family nudity in a July, 1975, *Redbook* article. Although Spock does not believe that an occasional accidental glimpse of a naked parent will be harmful to a child or that every child who sees his parents nude will suffer psychologically, he nevertheless advises parents not to let their children see them naked, at least on a regular basis. Why? Because Spock believes that family nudity could be sexually stimulating to the child and a factor in the development of various psychological problems such as frequent masturbation, sleeplessness, and school failure.

That this old-fashioned Freudian view has become accepted by many in our society is apparent. Dr. Joyce Brothers, in many respects a liberal psychologist, expressed a negative view about family nudity in her column in *Good Housekeeping* magazine. Asked whether it was healthy for parents to have taken their nine-month old baby into the tub with them, she stated that probably no great harm had been done—*thus far.* She adds that such family bathing should be discontinued: "Too much body contact and nudity in the home can create a kind of unconscious sexual frustration with which a young mind simply can't cope."

BODIES SHOULD NOT BE HIDDEN

Our own work and research has convinced us that this aspect of Freudian theory is based on invalid assumptions about bodies and sexuality. We believe that sometimes the hiding of the human body that takes place in families because of fears of sexual stimulation causes some of the very problems it is supposed to prevent—an overconcern with sexual parts and shock and/or disgust when these parts are finally seen.

Very small children have sexual feelings whether or not they see the genitals of the opposite sex. These feelings cannot be eliminated nor should they be. Like other strong emotions, these are not to be feared, only their repression or misdirection is to be feared. To help a child cope with his sexuality, a parent must be comfortable with and able to discuss the fact that the child *has* sexual feelings.

Why should a father have to hide his penis because it's bigger than his son's? The father doesn't hide his muscles, and they are also bigger and could cause envy. Nor does he hide the fact that he is taller. The comparative sizes of parts of children's and parents' bodies should be understood and coped with—not hidden.

Nor should a mother hide her genitals from her daughter. If a mother proudly allows her daughter to see genitals, pubic hair, and breasts, the daughter will look forward to becoming a woman.

A new breed of doctors, educators, and psychologists is challenging the idea that family nudity is damaging to children. Dr. Lee Salk wrote in his book *Preparing for Parenthood:*

> Although privacy for sexual intercourse seems appropriate, I see nothing wrong whatsoever in appearing nude before your children, who should become familiar with the human body, the differences between males and females, and the changes that occur in the body as a person matures.

Another expert, Dr. Sol Gordon, director of the Institute for Family Research and Education at Syracuse University, feels that the notion that parents might be seductive or overstimulating is an impediment that must be overcome if parents are to provide their children with needed sex information. Undressing in front of their young children or taking baths with them is something parents should try, Gordon says, "because it's a marvelous opportunity for parents to be 'askable' about their bodies."

A child with "askable" parents will find it easier to confide in them and ask about sexual feelings and bodily changes. An informed child will not have to "play doctor" in secret—his natural curiosity about bodies will be satisfied in the family situation. We are talking about more than sex education, of course. We are talking about *body education.*

Your home is the best place for your child to get a body education and you are the best person to give it to him. After all, if your child doesn't get a valid, realistic, sensible body education from you, he will likely get a distorted one from someone else. You can see that he obtains the kind of body knowledge that is a prerequisite to good health by giving him information about anatomy and physiology, answering questions about body parts and body functions in an open and matter-of-fact manner. And since a child's body image is related to how he thinks his parents feel about his body, physical affection is important. You can help him develop his sense of identity by respecting his feelings, including his sexual feelings. Only when a person knows what he feels and wants does he know who he is. You do have to teach him socially acceptable ways to express himself—but in the process, you need not suppress his body awareness or his ability to feel strong emotions.

One of the most important things you can do for your child's body education is not teach him to feel ashamed of his body.

However, sometimes even children raised to accept nudity and their bodies become more modest as they grow up. They may cover themselves up and want their parents to do so too. Many parents have noted that when children reach a more aware age, sometimes as early as between the ages of four and eight, going without clothing no longer seems so comfortable. Children at this age, especially those with older brothers and sisters, begin to tease younger children when they are naked. By going to school, by staying overnight at friends, and by other expansions of their world, children begin to learn that it is not considered permissible to take off their clothes around other people. At this uncomfortable point it may be easier for parents to avoid being nude in front of their children.

Another modest stage for many children occurs during the preadolescent and the teenage years. Whether or not less nudity is called for depends on the individual family. Los Angeles psychotherapist Evelyn Freeman and her psychologist husband, Albert Freeman, say of teenage nudity, "Any trauma is usually from puberty, not nudity. How can you suddenly say, 'Today you are thirteen; now you must suddenly stop taking off your clothes'? So much depends on what the teenager and his parents are feeling at the moment and how they are getting along."

The experiences of Los Angeles marriage counselors Jordan and Margie Paul, who have three children, tend to bear this out.

> "We don't make a big thing of it," says Mrs. Paul, "but when it is appropriate—when we are sleeping, when we get up in the morning, when we swim, and when the weather is warm—we take off our clothes.
>
> "Our children have decided, however, that they do not wish to be nude, at least in front of each other. Peer pressure, I think, is the main factor in their embarrassment with nudity right now, and Eric [nine years old] has asked us not to be nude when his friends are over. We respect that. However, Eric has no reluctance to being nude with Jordan and me. And those times, when we are nude together, are frequently the occasions when he asks questions about erections or masturbation or things like that."

As in many controversial areas different experts have reached different conclusions regarding family nudity. Our basic conclusion—based on our experience and that of hundreds of families we know about—is that family nudity promotes a lifelong attitude of body acceptance; body acceptance brings with it intellectual, psychological, and physical rewards. We think that family nudity is at least worth trying. If you would like to make family nudity part of your home environment, the following suggestions should help you do so in a totally natural way.

GUIDELINES FOR FAMILY NUDITY

There are three conditions for establishing the kind of atmosphere around the house in which every family member can feel comfortable with his own nakedness and the nakedness of others. These conditions are especially important for families with children past the toddler stage:

1. You must be comfortable with your own body.
2. You must be sensitive to your children's feelings about peer pressure and community standards.
3. You must allow your children to choose whether or not to undress.

Being Comfortable with Your Own Body

You can introduce nudity naturally into the family by beginning it yourself—by sleeping nude, by walking from the bathroom to the bedroom without clothes, by taking your time getting dressed, by making it clear to your child that if your bedroom door is open, it is all right for him to come in and talk, even if you are changing clothes. (You don't have to go to the toilet in front of your children, but if they are preschoolers, you might try leaving the bathroom door ajar sometimes. If your children intrude, convey the idea that toilet functions are a part of every person's daily life but that most people prefer privacy.) Just being in a variety of nude situations can help a parent gain body comfort and awareness.

You should delay family nudity until you are reasonably comfortable with your own sexuality and with your own feelings about nudity. Nudity is inappropriate if you feel more than a little uncomfortable about it. If it really is upsetting to you, if you are doing it only because you feel you should, not because you want to, don't do it.

A parent who feels uncomfortable about his own nudity and sexuality but is permitting his child to view his naked body for the child's "good" is sending as clear a message as if he thundered warnings about the sins of nudity. A parent who tells his child nudity is a wonderful experience that will free the child of all inhibitions but whose posture, facial expression, and tone of voice say it is really dirty or shameful is confusing his child and probably instilling some pretty negative attitudes about bodies in the process. First learn to feel comfortable about your own body and start listening more closely to your body "messages" and you will be less likely to transmit hidden negative messages to your children.

Being Sensitive to Children's Feelings about Others

Some parents worry that despite the body-education benefits family nudity may provide a child, he may suffer a form of social schizophrenia: his family does something that most other families consider taboo. But according to Dr. Norma Bernstein-Tarrow, associate professor in the Elementary Education Department at California State University at Long Beach, children are able to deal with the concept that one thing is acceptable to their parents and not acceptable to other people. Children are able to understand that by not going bare where neighbors can see them and by not talking about nudity to everyone, the family is not being hypocritical but is being considerate of the feelings of those with different beliefs. Being discreet is the way to avoid community disapproval of you and your children.

Arrange your house and yard for privacy, so that your activities cannot be viewed by neighbors. Parading nude in front of open windows or in an unfenced yard is obviously not the way to respect your neighbor's rights and sensibilities. (However, if you have fenced in your yard and keep your curtains drawn, you have done your part. Neighbors who have to climb fences or peer through curtain openings to see you are violating *your* rights.)

Certainly don't go bare in front of your children's friends or let the neighbor's children go nude in front of you or your children unless the parents of the children involved are present or have given you their permission.

Giving Children a Choice

It is best to allow children to make up their own minds about whether to be unclothed or not—and to allow them to change their minds. Tell them they have a choice of joining in or not—and that choice works for both parents and child. For example, you can say, "It's okay for you to sit out here on the deck without clothes, but I'm chilly and feel like leaving mine on." Or, "We're going to swim nude now, but you don't have to, if you don't want to."

The key word is *optional*. In a family where going bare is optional all members are free to wear as few clothes as they want, or none at all, without imposing their preferences on others and, equally important, without being subjected to put-downs.

Optional nudity means removing clothes is based on the idea of choice and appropriateness. It also includes the idea of privacy. For both parents and children a closed door should be a signal to other family members: "Leave me alone for a while." An open door means, "It's okay to come in and chat, even if I am changing clothes or taking a bath."

The concept of optional nudity made it simple, for example, for ten-year-old Peter to switch almost overnight from always wearing clothing to sometimes going bare. Peter's mother had remarried, and Peter's stepfather was in the habit of taking his clothes off around the house. Although Peter's mother also adopted the custom, they were unsure of how Peter would react, so they only took their clothes off when he was away or asleep. However, one sweltering night when his parents were sitting in the living room, minus clothing, watching television, Peter unexpectedly wandered downstairs. Seeing them cool and comfortable, and aware of his own hot, uncomfortable pajamas, Peter asked, "Do kids get to take their clothes off, too, or can only grownups do it?"

HOW TO BEGIN

No matter the age of your children, starting a policy of optional family nudity around the house can be easier than you might think *if* you pay attention to the guidelines we suggested. To facilitate the step from *never* going unclothed to *sometimes* going unclothed, we have provided some specific activities that will help you and your children achieve a sense of comfort with your own and each other's bodies. Not all of these activities involve nudity because before you can be comfortably unclad together, you have to learn to feel comfortable talking about, looking at, and touching each other's bodies.

1. Even in the most conservative communities the nakedness of infants and toddlers at home is not viewed with

alarm, and few modern child psychologists warn against parental nudity at this stage of a child's development. Here are some activities that should bring you and your baby benefits in the form of skin stimulation, motion, and closeness.

- Take him or her into the bathtub with you. The Japanese do this all the time, and although they have larger baths than we do, it could be managed in most American bathtubs. Your infant will get skin stimulation from you and from the water. Why should his bath consist of a lonely ritual in the Bathinette or sink?
- Gently rock your baby while in a hammock or rocking chair, holding his unclothed body next to your unclothed body. Next to skin contact, movement is the most important sensory experience your child requires at this point in his life.
- In situations where it is comfortable and practical for you and your baby to be unclothed for a period of time, carry him around while you do minor household tasks.

2. Since family nudity should not be forced, a good way to introduce it is in situations where it seems natural and appropriate, such as water-based activities. Dr. James Prescott believes that bathtime should be a family occasion: "The family bath should be used for socialization and relaxation," he says in *The Futurist* magazine, "and should provide a natural situation for children to learn about male-female differences." Obviously, a large bathtub, jacuzzi, or hot tub is needed if everyone is to fit. This activity is easily started with your children while they are still preschoolers.

3. If you want to teach younger children that parts of the body are mentionable, or teach older children anatomical names, or teach younger and older children to feel comfortable about touching all parts of their bodies, the children's game "Simon Says" is helpful. "Simon" can tell the children to touch their knees, their shoulders, the tips of their fingers, their vulvae, breasts, or penises (or, for older children, their clavicles, tibiae, or metacarpals). (For body coordination exercises, "Simon" can tell the children to touch elbows to knees, fingers to ears, and so forth.)

4. Families can learn to become more comfortable about the idea of family nudity by looking at pictures of naked bodies and talking about them. You can ask your

young children to draw pictures of their own bodies, clothed and unclothed, and discuss the drawings with them, paying attention to words they use to describe the various body parts and to body parts they overemphasize or leave out.

Keep magazines with pictures of nude bodies around your house. When your children are looking at the pictures, initiate a discussion about nudity and bodies. While this may seem threatening to you or your children at first, feelings—about nudity or anything else—are only threatening if you never discuss or learn to understand them. Within your own family circle you can develop the ability to talk openly about your feelings. In fact, in a body-prejudiced society, the home is probably the only place where your children will have a chance to learn to express their feelings and accept their bodies.

5. Earlier we told you how vital touch is to your children's development and good health. Here is a suggestion: Try a bedtime massage instead of bedtime story. (It's surprising how tense even little children's bodies can feel at the end of the day.) Parents can even ask their kids for a pre-dinner massage instead of having a pre-dinner cocktail. Letting the kids rub your back and neck can sometimes do more for you than a martini.

Remember that the *way* you touch communicates your feelings. When you want your child to stop dawdling at the supermarket, the smile on your face may fool the other shoppers, but the hurry-up shove you give him says you are irritated. It will be more difficult for him to accept and enjoy his body if your irritation is frequently conveyed to him by the way you touch him. All family members need a chance to talk about touching—to freely express their feelings about *how* they are being touched by other family members. Twelve-year-old Johnny may like playful wrestling with his dad but may object to being pinned down so he can't move. Grandmother may want more healthy, hearty, spontaneous hugs from the rest of the family instead of the hurried pats which deprive her of the body contact she needs.

In fact, two-generation sleeping arrangements may be desirable. For example, one widowed grandmother discovered—when asked to share a bed with one of the kids during a family emergency—that a warm body cuddled up next to her at night gives her a sense of comfort and enables her to fall asleep. A small child who goes to bed earlier than the rest of the family might feel less lonely and left out if he knows that on some nights someone will join him later. Though most Americans believe it is healthier for children to sleep alone, warm contact with another body might be far more desirable for some children.

6. Body contracts may help family members reinforce the new type of behavior the family is trying out. In addition, the contracts help family members learn better habits of caring for their bodies—of doing things that are not only good for them but that give them pleasure. The contracts can be verbal or written; many kids love the drama of drawing up legal-type agreements. A contract has two parts: In the first part, the person making the contract states several realistic goals for his own body such as taking a walk twice a week, getting a massage once a month, exercising ten minutes a day. In the second part, he states things he is going to do for the bodies of the people in his family—hug them upon greeting and parting, serve less fattening foods, give someone a "body compliment" every day. The contracts work better if a family member can get another to help him reach his own body goals. For example, mother may want to swim at least once a week. She can make a body contract with a family member to go swimming with her and in return she will do something good for that person's body (a massage, a low-calorie but delicious meal, or chauffeuring services to a dance or exercise class).

7. Body games can lead to one of our previously mentioned promises—body joy. These games are listed in Chapter 14. They are absolutely guaranteed to provoke a lot of laughter, which is probably the first step towards achieving body joy.

Chapter 9
Going Bare with Your Sexual Partner

> The people we see who have sexual problems tend to be uptight about their bodies and about nudity. Almost always they wear something to bed. They wear clothes to bed even in the summertime when it is hot. There is practically never any skin contact.... Often sex is restricted to night, in the dark, under the covers. These kinds of things put a lot of prohibitions on being spontaneous and free with each other.
>
> Dr. William Hartman,
Center for Marital and Sexual Studies,
Long Beach, California

Can you talk about all the parts of the body and its functions frankly and without embarrassment? Are you and your partner able to look freely at each other's bodies in both sexual and nonsexual situations? How much do you really know about where and how your partner likes to be touched?

Even in our age of sexual liberation, surprisingly few people have positive answers to these questions. According to Richard Littrell, marriage counselor at the American Institute of Family Relations in Los Angeles, among the people he works with, discomfort with the body is common:

> My experience has been that the vast majority of my clients are uncomfortable with nudity; most of them do

not see each other in the nude regularly—you know, their backs are turned or they are making a dash for the bathroom to take a shower or dress or whatever. And many times their sex becomes one of those fast operations that seems to say, "Let's get this over as quick as we can because I don't want to discover too much about you or you about me."

HIDING YOUR BODY FROM YOUR PARTNER

Many couples limit the amount of body exposure they allow each other, without realizing how much they are reducing their sexual pleasure and other aspects of their relationship. A woman may be loving and open, yet refuse to make love with the lights on because she has such a negative picture of her body that she is convinced the sight of it during sex will turn her lover off. A man may be verbally uninhibited on the subject of sex, but always wear pajamas to bed, removing only the bottoms during intercourse. We know a nurse who claims nudity is no big deal to her (she "bathes naked people every working day of her life") yet she always wants to wear a filmy negligee or a shorty nightgown while making love because, she says, "I feel more sexually exciting when wearing something."

People hide their bodies from their partners for a variety of reasons, and often are not aware of the real reasons. Although they may claim various excuses, the two major underlying reasons are a negative body image and shame about body functions.

Although you and your lover may encounter each other in some of the most intimate of ways, you may be as shy about discussing certain subjects with each other as you would be with strangers. Just as the Victorians believed some subjects "too embarrassing to mention," most of us do, too, namely body faults, body odors, and sexual secretions. Very few couples ever discuss what they regard to be their body's major faults. They hope that by not calling attention to the fault, their partner won't "notice it." But then they act as if the partner had noticed it.

Not liking some part (or all) of your body and feeling compelled to use clothes or darkness to disguise or conceal it can create the very rejection you fear. A woman who is—or just thinks she is—flat-chested (and therefore unfeminine) may not want to undress in front of her partner—and as a result he may feel cheated and resent her behavior. Although he may never articulate it, a man who believes his penis is abnormally small (and thus that he is not masculine enough) may try to keep that part of his anatomy covered, and after sex always put his shorts or pajamas back on right away. Though he is unable to tell his wife he feels inferior about his penis size, she may sense he is uncomfortable about something and, not knowing what, may fear it is something about her.

A friend once said he used to think that being intimate with a woman meant you were able to have oral-genital contact with her, but then he discovered that the true test was: "Could you fart in front of her without embarrassment?" While we are certainly not suggesting that breaking wind will *create* intimacy, the fact remains that this natural body function should not be a taboo subject for sexually intimate couples.

Body odors are another commonly taboo subject. A husband may fail to respond to his wife's sexual overtures because he feels sweaty from working in the garden and is afraid his odor will offend her. He may never discover that she finds the smell exciting. In our society both the smells themselves and the subject of smells have been covered up. Dr. Harold Greenwald, professor of psychology at United States International University in San Diego, California, says:

> As very little kids, one of the worst things you can say to someone is "you stink." We are so afraid of offending that breath sprays, deodorants, and vaginal sprays have tremendous sales. There are women who won't go to bed with a man if there is no shower available, because they are fearful they will offend him. And it is true that one of the biggest lacks of communication and one of the greatest turn-offs many men and women have reported to me in sex is the odor—not just the kind that

emanates from unwashed genitals but the odor someone has when you kiss them.

Greenwald says that, without realizing it, people frequently are attracted to someone primarily on the basis of the way they smell. Body odors cause powerful reactions, particularly the odors of a sexual partner, and human behavior is much more dependent upon smell than most people realize. Body aromas can be a natural aphrodisiac. People need to let their partners know what body smells they like and people need to be able to talk openly about odors in general.

Another undiscussed subject between many intimate partners is sexual secretions such as semen and menstrual blood. A wife who feels passionate during her menstrual period may be afraid to initiate sex for fear the presence of blood will be repulsive to her husband. She is also likely to fear talking about it. A man who always jumps right up after intercourse, brings his wife a towel to dry herself, and then takes a shower may believe he is being thoughtful. However, his wife may feel insulted, thinking he wants to wash off her vaginal secretions immediately. If she is too shy to talk about it, the situation persists. Many couples are victims of their own conspiracy of silence concerning things "too embarrassing to mention."

Just as hiding your feelings about body subjects can have a negative influence on your intimacy and your relationship with your partner, so does hiding your body. The ability of partners to be comfortably nude around each other at times when they don't want or expect sex is important for those who want a genuinely good sex life. Your ability to give freely of your body during sex is directly related to how comfortable you are with your naked body and with the naked body of your partner—all the time. The more body freedom you have, the more feelings of satisfaction and fulfillment you will have in sex.

Expanding your comfort level with your own and your partner's nude body may open up a whole new dimension of closeness, intimacy, and satisfaction. But getting to this level of comfort isn't always easy. You may be willing to use nonsexual nudity to increase your body freedom and enhance your sex life, but what do you do if your partner isn't ready?

HOW TO GET YOUR PARTNER TO GO BARE

There are three conditions for establishing the kind of atmosphere in which your partner can feel comfortable about being undressed:

1. You need to demonstrate comfort with your own body.
2. You should give frequent praise of his or her body.
3. You must be patient with your partner.

Demonstrating Comfort with Your Own Body

Whenever you casually undress in front of your partner, walk from the bathroom to the bedroom without clothes, or sleep nude, you are showing that you feel comfortable with your body. You are showing that nudity is natural and that the sex act does not necessarily have to follow every exposure of your own or your partner's body. Showing affection while nude can be pleasurable, emotionally nourishing, and a tender way of establishing a habit of *non*erotic touching.

A way to start is by going to bed nude and snuggling with your partner, giving him or her skin-to-skin contact before going to sleep at night and before getting up in the morning. It may help persuade him or her to learn to sleep nude. Marriage counselor Jordan Paul describes what happened when he decided to adopt his wife's custom of sleeping without clothes:

> I had never stopped to realize how ridiculous it was to get undressed only to get dressed again to go to bed and if we had sex, to get undressed again and then dressed again afterward. So I shed all nighttime attire and discovered that the intrusion of nightclothes had been cutting me off from one of the most pleasurable experiences I have ever had. The feeling of Margie's softness and warmth throughout the night is comforting and sensual to me. Now, our orientation toward bedtime is

not to go to sleep right away but to hold each other and be affectionate.

A husband who thinks that being naked is necessarily an invitation to sex, and who attempts to initiate sex whenever his wife is bare, will inevitably condition her against taking her clothes off if she isn't in the mood for sex.

Giving Frequent Verbal Reinforcement

What you say about your partner's body and how you treat him when he is nude will have a great deal to do with how he feels about his body and the amount of nudity he will be comfortable with in the relationship.

If a wife says "Your stomach's hanging out. I thought you said you were going on a diet" or if a husband says "Your breasts look like two fried eggs," the recipients of such remarks will tend to stay covered up. What we need is reinforcement about nude bodies, especially from those we love the most. And we need it all our lives, as our bodies change and as our relationships change.

One of the nicest and least expensive gifts you can give is a compliment about your partner's body. In *Free to Love*,* Jordan Paul describes the pleasure he felt when his wife came into the bathroom while he was shaving and remarked that she loved to look at his body:

> "How come you never said that to me before?"
>
> "I don't know. It's obvious that you have a nice body. I guess I was embarrassed to say it."
>
> "But I've never felt good about my body. My chest is too thin, and I'm not muscular enough."
>
> "I've never liked men with super-muscular builds."
>
> . . .
>
> I knew Margie didn't dislike my body, but to hear that she loved it made me feel terrific. I looked in the mirror. It really was nice. I wanted to hear more. "What else do you like about my body?" I asked.

---

*From *Free to Love*, by Jordan & Margaret Paul. Los Angeles: J.P. Tarcher, Inc., copyright © 1975 by Jordan and Margaret Paul.

Talking with your partner is a vital step. Reinforcement does not only mean that you say good things about the beautiful parts of your partner's body. Relationships go beyond what the eye sees; one can say "I like to feel the warmth of your body," "I like the way you smell," "I enjoy touching you when you don't have clothes on," "I like the way you taste," or any number of things that don't compare your intimate partner's body to idealized forms—forms that we've been taught to measure bodies by.

Being Patient with Your Partner

When you and your lover disagree about what is a desirable amount of nudity—and about when and where and for whom—tolerance is necessary. And patience. There is no hurry. The shedding of clothing will not automatically bring you instant happiness or a better sex life. However, the way you talk about nudity can cause your mate unhappiness and thus can hamper your sex life.

Explore the issue when your partner is in a *good mood* and *willing* to talk openly. Don't try to change your partner's mind—to get him to do what you want and to see things *your* way—instead listen to and understand him. Try to become aware of how your partner is feeling and why he feels that way. Ask him to do the talking exercise described next, explaining that talking is all you will expect.

Do not imply that your partner is behind the times, uptight, uninformed, or stubborn. Do not suggest there is anything wrong with his feelings, fears, fantasies, wishes, or opinions. For example, if she says, "I just don't feel right when I walk around nude," recognize she is just telling you about her discomfort—not saying that she will *never* feel right about it or that there is anything wrong with you because you like it. Let her talk. She is making a gift of her feelings at the moment, and if you put her down by saying "That's really a dumb way to feel—the trouble is, you are just inhibited," she may not make you another gift. Don't try to talk her out of her discomfort, because you love her and would like to free her of it or because you are angry and feel hemmed in by it.

BODY LIBERATION ACTIVITIES

The exercises that follow will enhance your sexual relationship and help you achieve greater body freedom.

Talking Exercise

If you and your partner are interested in enhancing your sexual relationship through increasing your sense of body comfort, here is a talking exercise you can do together. Find magazines that feature full frontal nudity (*Playboy*, *Penthouse*, *Viva*, *Playgirl*, and others) and look at them together. Talk about the way the pictures of both your own and the opposite sex make you feel. Answering some of the following questions can sometimes trigger new ideas and insights.

    1. How do the pictures of persons of my own sex make me feel about my body?
    2. If I looked like that person, what do I fantasize my life would be like?
    3. What fantasies do I have about the person in the magazine of the opposite sex?
    4. How would that person feel about me?

Looking and Touching

Here are some activities that involve looking at and touching each other's bodies, to be done with your partner at a time when you do *not* intend to have sex. Though they will help you increase your comfort level with your own and your partner's body—a worthwhile achievement—they are meant to be play, not work. Have fun with them.

    1. Undress each other in the dark. Make an agreement with one another not to talk until you are all through and to touch one another in an exploratory, not an erotic way.

While you are touching, pretend you are blind and do not know your partner. Imagine you are trying to get to know your partner's body well enough to recognize it by touch in the future, that you are trying to get a sense of what kind of person he is and trying to let him know what kind of person you are.

Afterwards share as much as you can with one another about what was going on in your minds during this procedure.

2. Give your partner a bath—preferably in water to which you've added bubble bath, bath oil beads, or some other product to make the process feel luxurious and delightful to the senses. Let your partner bathe you on a different day. One person should have full attention without the feeling that he has to give anything back. Make this a caring experience—not a sexually provocative one. Take total responsibility for your partner's body. Wash him thoroughly as you would a baby, and with your touch and look try to convey that you find his body pleasing to you.

When you are through, help him out of the tub and gently dry him. Pat on body powder or after-bath lotion. Wrap him in a soft robe or big beach towel and lie beside him on a bed or on a floor with a thick carpet. Be quiet and look into one another's eyes for a while—and then, when you are ready, talk softly with one another about the thoughts and feelings you had and are having.

3. Take a shower together. Wash each other, shampoo each other's hair, and dry each other. Make this a playful, not an erotic experience. As you soap and rinse and dry one another's bodies, play with mounds of soapsuds, the water, the sponge or washcloth, the towel, and each other's hair and body parts.

4. Stand in front of a mirror together without any clothes on. A full length mirror is best. Look at each other and at yourself and try to get a sense of how you feel about the two persons you are looking at—as individuals and as a couple—and how you feel about looking at their bodies. Take turns and, one person at a time, feel your *own* body all over while the other partner watches. The partner who is watching should observe and later reveal what parts the other avoids touching, what parts he seems to enjoy touching, and his apparent moods and feelings during this exercise.

This exercise presents an opportunity to discuss how each feels about specific parts of his body and to give one another reassurance. Although a person doesn't have to like all parts of his body equally well, if your partner has some part he really hates, it should be brought to his attention and discussed. He might want to ask himself what effect the hate of that part is having on his life. It could also be helpful to assure him that he is lovable anyway. If there is some part that he thinks is just perfect, you can rejoice with him but assure him that he'd still be lovable if that part wasn't so great.

5. While you and your partner are both naked take turns saying ten things you like about each other's body. Alternate so that each gives one compliment and touches that part, then the other gives a compliment and touches that part. For example, one might say, "I like your hairy chest" and then stroke it. The other could say, "I like the dimples on your bottom" and then pat it.

6. Have one partner lie or sit in a comfortable position, nude, while the other touches him all over his body. The one who is being touched should close his eyes and focus his awareness on where and how he is being touched and indicate the sort of touch he likes by calling out numbers, using a scale from one to ten. For example, he might say, "That was a five" when his partner touches him somewhere. The partner should then try different kinds of touch to see if he can bring the rating up. If he cannot bring the rating up, it may indicate the person is just not as interested in being touched in that particular place as in some other. Obviously, a ten rating indicates a favorite place is being touched in just the right way. Be sure to talk with one another afterward to recall and verify your partner's favorite places and favorite ways of being touched.

7. The purpose of this exercise is threefold: to help partners learn to receive pleasure from each other without feeling as though they must hurry and give something back, to learn how to direct each other's touching, and to discover the many ways of getting pleasure while giving it. A couple may do this exercise together many different times. It gets better every time.

There is a giver and a receiver. Partners take turns playing each part, going through three segments of the technique and then reversing roles. The person who is to be the receiver decides what part of his body he wants touched and what parts he wants left alone. For example: "I'd like you to touch my upper back but do not touch my buttocks."

Use an egg timer or some other device to time the activity which takes place in three three-minute sections:

Step 1. The giver focuses his complete and undivided attention on the part specified by the receiver, trying to give it as much pleasure through touching as he possibly can—and at the same time enjoying himself in the process.

The receiver is not to react at all—show no expression, say nothing, just lie back and enjoy.

Step 2. The giver is again to give pleasure to that part by being playful, tender, or whatever he thinks will give both partners pleasure. However this time the receiver is to indicate his reactions—but *without* words. He can use signs, grunts, moans, smiles, frowns, hums, purrs, etc. This goes on for three minutes also.

Step 3. The giver is to focus attention on the same spot, but is to do only what the receiver asks for in words. For example, "Please rub my shoulder harder," "Run your fingers down my spine," etc. At the end of three minutes, the giver and receiver reverse positions and the process is repeated.

When each partner has had a turn in each position, they talk about what happened, how they felt, what they particularly liked, and what bothered them. If they have any insights, they share them and discuss possible changes in their ways of touching one another or of making love based on these insights and newly discovered feelings.

FAMILIARITY BREEDS PLEASURE

A common worry is that of overfamiliarity—that if you and your partner get totally familiar with each other's bodies, there will be loss of sexual interest, you will begin taking each other for granted, the "magic" will go out of your relationship. This may be true for some couples, but we don't believe it will happen in most cases. We are convinced that increasing a person's comfort with his own and his partner's body parts and processes and with nudity (in both sexual and non-sexual situations) will enhance, not detract from, his sex life.

Evidence that nudity can and frequently does improve one's sex life comes from a study involving three thousand people by sociologists William Hartman and Marilyn Fithian, directors of the Center for Marital and Sexual Studies in Long Beach, California. They reported that nudity not only enhanced the sexual happiness of the majority of nudist married couples but also that many non-nudists who attended camps reported a subsequent change for the better in their sexual behavior. Learning to be comfortably nude in the presence of others apparently gives a person a sense of self-acceptance. Observing that nonorgasmic women tend to have a negative self-image, Hartman and Fithian designed a body-image improvement technique that requires an individual to be nude and to look at, touch, and talk about his body while looking in a mirror in the presence of both a male and a female therapist. This technique is a basic part of any treatment of sexually dysfunctioning couples at the Center for Marital and Sexual Studies.

Another powerful technique developed by Hartman and Fithian is the sexological examination. They devised it after noting that most people believe their sex organs are deficient in some way and usually compare theirs unfavorably with others. Unlike a medical examination, which is concerned with discovering disease, the purpose of the sexological examination is to discover what is right about a person's sex organs and how to use them for greater sexual pleasure. The client, as well as the examiner, looks at, touches, and talks about these private parts. The examination is conducted in a relaxed manner by a professional person of the opposite sex who is wearing street clothes. (A therapist of the opposite sex always takes a client's sexual history and does the sexological examination to accustom the person taking the exam to a situation in which one looks at sexual parts and talks about sexual activities with a member of the opposite sex.) Both scientific and colloquial terms are used and a light banter usually develops between examiner and client.

Throughout both procedures, Hartman and Fithian do everything possible to make certain the client will experience himself as a human being with feelings as well as sex organs, rather than as an object under a microscope.

If the client wishes, his or her mate may join in exploring the sex organs. Fithian thinks this participation is important: A husband's interest in his wife's genitals helps eliminate feelings of shame and disgust. A wife's interest helps reassure a man who may be insecure about the size of his penis or the appearance of his testicles.

Even couples who have what they consider a satisfactory sex life can benefit from the basic Hartman-Fithian techniques of looking at, talking about, and touching their own and their partners' nude bodies. Here, for instance, is what happened when a newly married couple in their early thirties, whom we'll call Kathleen and Bill, underwent the sexological. Kathleen is blonde, attractive, and after six months of marriage (the second for both of them) more in love with Bill than she was when they married. She didn't perceive herself as needing help with either body image or sexual functioning, but Bill believed she did not see her body realistically. Although his approval enabled her to be nude in front of him, she still thought of her body as "grotesque." Bill's approval could not, by itself, change her self-concept because, like many people, she tended to discount compliments from a person who loved her.

Kathleen's negative self-image began when, as a child, it became obvious to her that her parents were not happy with the way she looked. She recalled her mother excusing Kathleen's appearance to an acquaintance with, "Yes, Kathleen is going to be getting her braces off soon. And she is on a diet. Of course, she doesn't *always* wear glasses." Kathleen's first husband didn't help when, the first week they were married, he came up behind her when she was nude and said, "The backs of your legs look like washboards; they have funny little dents in them." After that she hated being undressed around him and began covering her body more and more, eliminating shorts from her wardrobe.

When Bill heard that we were looking for people to participate in Hartman and Fithian's sexological and body image procedures for research purposes, he thought that this sort of program would be helpful for Kathleen. He talked it over with her and she agreed, more to please Bill than because she thought she needed help.

During the first part of Kathleen's sexological examination, Bill was not in the room. This is part of the Hartman and Fithian structure to protect the wife in case they discover any problems that might embarrass her or which a husband might later, through ignorance or malice, use against her. Were they to discover weak vaginal muscles, for example (a common finding in many women), they would not want the husband to say, "No wonder we have lousy sex; you have weak vaginal muscles!" As Kathleen lay on the examining table, Hartman looked for any physical problems that might lessen her or Bill's pleasure during intercourse—such as clitoral adhesions.

By helping her go through a series of body explorations and carefully inspecting parts of herself she had never seen before, she began to discover her sensitivity and response patterns and find new pleasure areas. Using a mirror, Kathleen was able to inspect her own genital area, even to see inside her vagina. Like a travel guide, Hartman combined a lecture on female anatomy with remarks on her particular anatomy:

> Here's the labia majora and these are the labia minora. In about half of the women their minora are longer than their majora. You're one of those. Now let's look at your clitoris. See that? The prepuce, this fold like a foreskin, is probably adhered there. In terms of orgasmic response, it could help to free it up a little. The urethra, through which you pass urine, is right there. What I'm touching is your cervix. Your uterus is in a normal position. Now tighten your vaginal muscles. Make believe you are going to urinate and you have to stop it. You have pretty good vaginal muscles, but I'm going to give you some exercises to make them tighter.

Then Bill was admitted to the room, and told how to use the plastic speculum so that he could peer inside. Gently slipping the lighted speculum through her genital folds, he guided it into her vagina and gazed with fascination. Bill had many questions: "Is that the uterus?" "Where does the sperm go?" "Does a baby really come out of that tiny cervix?" Bill was delighted with the opportunity to get a first-hand education.

Hartman then instructed Bill on how to do the "vaginal caress," which consisted of putting his index finger into her vagina, with its tip touching a ring of tissue barely inside the opening, and moving the fingertip from the uppermost "12 o'clock" position to "1 o'clock," "2 o'clock," and so on, asking Kathleen which places were most pleasurable. Hartman also told them of a pleasurable exercise consisting of Bill's going around all the "clock" positions as Kathleen instructed "faster," "heavier," "slower," etc.

Following the sexological examination, Bill was asked to leave the room again, and Kathleen was led through a series of body-image improvement techniques. Standing in front of a three-way mirror with her back to Hartman and Fithian, she was asked to touch and talk about every part of her anatomy, starting with her head. She described how each part looked to her and how she felt about it. Although she is a pretty woman with small shoulders, firm breasts, a well-defined waistline, and rounded (but not fat) hips and thighs, that was not what she saw. She was not too unkind to the upper part of her body ("I have nice square shoulders. My arms are a little too fleshy in here and that bothers me. I never wear anything that doesn't have sleeves. I have nice, soft skin...") but when she got to what she called her "problem area" the interchange with Hartman went like this:

Kathleen: This is my problem area, my hips. They are just horrible.

Hartman: How do you feel about being a good fleshy hippie?

Kathleen: I hate it. I hate to wear a bathing suit and let people see me. If I wore a bikini, they could see the whole thing. My broken skin lines and all those dimply fat marks. Sure leaves a lot to be desired... [My legs] are grotesque. I'm ashamed of them. I don't want anybody to see them... Bill thinks they are okay, though.

Hartman: Sounds like Bill is talking you into a lot of good things. Too bad you couldn't talk yourself into them independently. Look at that woman in the mirror. Give her a rating from zero to 100—about how do you feel about that woman.

Kathleen: (Smiling) I'll give her a good 75.

Later, Bill was given his sexological exam, with Fithian checking his genitals (and nipples) for sensitivity, looking for any conditions that might inhibit sexual enjoyment, and making suggestions for things he could do to increase his or Kathleen's pleasure. Kathleen was asked to take his genitals—first his penis, then his testicles—in her hands while he was told to instruct her as to how firmly he liked them held and how and where he liked to be touched.

Bill also went through a body image improvement procedure, but saw his body much more positively than Kathleen had seen hers. He gave himself a body acceptance rating of 95 percent.

To many people, the idea of inspecting their partner's genitals may seem too clinical and a certain killer of romance. They prefer to retain an air of mystery and they certainly have that option. But for Bill and Kathleen, the sexological examination and the body-image work not only changed their attitudes but their actual behavior in regard to nudity and sex. For Bill, witnessing Kathleen's sexological examination was the most significant part of the experience. As he said later, "The vagina had always been a sort of mysterious zone to me; a place I had never seen and didn't really know that much about. Looking at it and sharing my feelings about it heightened my awareness."

For Kathleen, the most significant part of the experience was the body-image work: "Dr. Hartman didn't know me and had no sexual interest in me, yet he had many positive things to say about my body. It was beautiful to hear. I waited for thirty years to hear something good about my body from someone who didn't love me or want to make love to me."

Kathleen, who had never really been comfortable walking around the house with nothing on, even when alone, became able to take great enjoyment in her own nudity. Both were freed of inhibitions they hadn't known they had. Their lives became more playful, more adventurous, and more intimate.

YOUR OWN SEXOLOGICAL EXAMINATION

If there is a sex clinic in your area or doctors or psychologists listed as sexual therapists, inquire if they are familiar with the sexological examination and are willing to do it as a separate technique without your having to go through a whole course of therapeutic procedures (or you might want to go through the whole course). If the people you contact can't do what you want, ask them for a referral to someone who will.

Or when a wife goes for her regular yearly or semi-yearly gynecological examination, she can request that her husband be permitted to observe the examination and be told about what is taking place. Some doctors may resist this idea as being too time-consuming, unprofessional, or embarrassing. Doctors are used to talking about pathology, not sexual pleasure. Many have had little experience with nude bodies. The cover-up sheet used in examinations may protect the doctor more than the patient. Even if your doctor is a gynecologist or an obstetrician, he may not be familiar with the sensitivity in the walls of the vagina, the appearance of tissue that indicates a lack of tone, and the kinds of exercises that can be done to increase sexual pleasure. Hartman and Fithian, who give six-week training courses to professionals, find medical and nonmedical clients equally in need of training.

If you meet resistance, don't give up. The trend in medicine is slowly changing—at the insistence of patients who want to be let in on what is going on in their own bodies. If you let your doctor know you are interested in educating yourself about your body, he just may cooperate. Husbands in the examining room should be no more unusual than husbands in the delivery room.

You may want to take charge of your own sexological examination. With the aid of a good anatomy book, a plastic speculum, a flashlight, and a mirror, you and your partner can conduct a do-it-yourself sexological. (This is an extension of the feminist idea of medical self-help groups in which women examine themselves and each other.) Learning to look at and identify parts of your own and your partner's body is no more complex than learning about your oral cavity—and it is a lot more interesting. However, we suggest a couple of preliminaries:

1. It is a good idea for the woman to get a vaginal examination by her physician before beginning the sexological.

2. Exercise caution in using a speculum. Plastic speculums can be purchased cheaply but they can damage tissue if

not properly used. Have someone (your doctor, a nurse, a laboratory technician, someone at a feminist center) show you the correct way to use it. It is not difficult to learn how.

PART TWO
BEYOND BODY TABOOS

Chapter 10
Going Bare with Others

> In this country the human body has only recently and partially come to light. Its discovery has taken us by surprise, and many still regard it with suspicion. For historical and emotional reasons in our society the naked body is believed to be incomplete—a body minus clothes. It is the packaged product that we take for the man and the woman.
>
> Bernard Rudofsky,
> *The Unfashionable Human Body*

If you are still with us you have come a long way toward achieving body pride. You have become more knowledgeable about and comfortable with your body. You probably feel more natural going bare around your family. In this second half of the book we are going to ask you to take a new look at one of the strongest remaining body taboos—the taboo against revealing your entire body to those not of your own family.

Social nudity is disturbing to most people, and you will probably find yourself instantly on guard. Most people resist the idea of disrobing for anything besides bathing and sex. After all, they may say, what can you do unclothed that you can't do with a swimsuit on? Nudity can be embarrassing, even dangerous, they say, because it could result in sexual arousal—in oneself, one's spouse, or others (and here the mind can become quite imaginative, producing pictures of infidelity, rape, group sex, arrest, and disgrace).

Because most people have strong ideas on the subject, let us first state what we are *not* going to try to make you do.

We are not going to try to turn you into a full-time "nudist." We are not going to try to get you into an uncomfortable situation where you have to cope with leers, voyeurism, unwanted caresses, propositions, swinging, homosexuality, and so on (it is symptomatic of the confusion in our society about the unclothed body that all these associations even arise).

This is a consciousness-raising book and we are asking you to rethink some attitudes you may have toward your body and the bodies of others. We are suggesting some body-liberating experiences that include the occasional shedding of clothing in the presence of others under safe and appropriate circumstances. Let us describe the benefits.

Self-acceptance. The major premise of this book is that your body is you. Not liking your body is tantamount to not liking yourself. Discovering that other people can look at your body as it is—undisguised and unconcealed—and accept you *as you are* is a vital step in accepting yourself. Dr. Herbert Otto believes that full acceptance of one's body can come about only through group nudity: "It isn't enough to own your body and to feel good about your body in the privacy of your home. It's when you can accept your body in the company of others who are not your family that your deepest sense of self-acceptance can be nourished."

Satisfying your curiosity about other people's bodies. Most of us only get to compare our own bodies to the beautiful ones we see in magazines and have little idea about what the average nude body looks like. To learn more about our own bodies and know how we really compare to others, we have to have the opportunity to see other average, naked human bodies—to realize what a wide range of acceptable sizes, shapes, colors, and ages there are.

It is natural to be curious about what other people look like without clothes. And social nudity, in a nonsexual context, is a way to fulfill this curiosity.

Freedom from social role-playing. We use clothing to make a statement about ourselves, to tell others we are a certain kind of person—chic, hip, rebellious, scholarly, wealthy, sexy, liberal, conservative, whatever. At a nudist camp or nude beach, people seem to shed their social roles. It becomes impossible to hide behind expensive clothing. Freedom from role restraints is one reason people experience such a sense of well-being on nude beaches.

THE RELATIVISM OF MODESTY

While shedding social roles now and then is unquestionably liberating, chances are many people feel that nudity around others violates a basic aspect of human nature—something we call "modesty." Almost all of the arguments against social nudity center on the idea that exposure of the sexual organs is to be avoided—and may even be morally wrong—because it creates sexual arousal in a member of the opposite sex. Therefore as long as a female hides her breasts and sexual organs in a few patches of cloth called a bikini or a man covers his organs in a very brief pair of swim trunks, they both still remain within the limits of modesty. This viewpoint, however, is the result of our cultural upbringing rather than our innate biological destiny.

Anthropologist Ruth Benedict noted that dress did not originate as much because people were concerned about others seeing their sexual parts as because of their desire to look better—their *vanity*. Apparently man's own bare body affects him as a blank canvas affects an artist. From prehistory on, humans have painted, decorated, and hung objects on their bodies in a number of ways and for a number of purposes, including status, a desire to look more attractive, and sexual selection. Some higher primates such as chimpanzees have been observed hanging objects on their bodies and prancing around seeking attention and admiration from the other animals.

Different societies at various times in history have been modest about different parts of the body. Females in both nineteenth-century China and seventeenth-century Spain were modest about their feet. In fact, during the reign of Philip II of Spain, carriages had a specially fitted mechanism that could be lowered to hide the feet of women as they disembarked. When it was suggested that women's dresses be shortened so they would raise less dust, husbands said they would rather see their wives dead than share the sight of their feet with other men.

In the last century, Victorian morality permitted formal dresses that displayed cleavage, but forbade the displaying of bare arms.

Until the 1930s, Comanche Indian males felt "indecent" if they ventured out in public without wearing their G-strings, even though they might be covered from head to foot with American store-bought pants and shirts.

Present-day Arab peasant women have been known to throw their skirts over their heads when caught out in the fields without a veil because it is immodest to show their faces.

In Japan the nape of the neck used to be considered an erotic part of the body that a woman only revealed for the purpose of arousing a man.

The Japanese attitude toward the **naked human body** in some respects tends to be even more negative than ours. Until recently, the sight of the naked body was not acceptable in traditional art and even Japanese pornography pictured the lovers dressed. A few years ago, when *Playboy* magazine began featuring pictures of nudes with pubic hair, all vestiges of *chimo* (Japanese for "shameful hair") had to be airbrushed out before the magazines could be distributed in Japan. Yet in other respects the Japanese are most accepting of nudity. The communal bath is a case in point. Out of necessity (70 percent of all homes in Tokyo don't have baths), love of cleanliness, and sociability, the custom of the communal bath (there are 2500 in Tokyo alone) and nude, mixed-sex bathing prevails. Jack Seward, author of *The Japanese*, witnessed about 150 teenage boys and girls splashing around together at a communal bath in Hokkaido. They were on a school-sponsored excursion and the male and female teachers chaperoning them were not "shirking their duties. All of them were right there in the bath with their charges—and just as bare."

Some clothing historians claim that clothing is far sexier than nudity. James Laver, author of *Modesty in Dress*, says, "If complete nudity were common, we should probably become seasonal in our impulses, like the animals. Our characteristic *permanent* eroticism is kept alive by clothes." And this eroticism is activated by style changes which result in emphasis of first one and then another part of the body.

Today the female bosom, partly exposed in low-cut or see-through dresses, is considered sexy. Legs are also considered sexy, though somewhat less so than a few years back: Their "erotic capital" (a term devised by Laver) has been lowered through over-exposure.

At certain periods in history, men have also built up erotic capital. Early in the fifteenth century, males wore clinging tights which extended up to the waistline, and which not only showed off the legs but also clearly accentuated the genitals. Men also wore doublets which were so short that bending over exposed the wearer's "breeks (breeches) and what is inside them to those standing behind."

The Church, concerned about masculine modesty and failing through fines and other punishments to stop the wearing of clinging hose and short doublets, ordered the placement of a piece of material over the genitals. This covering, usually made of leather, developed into the codpiece or braguette, a pouch that fit over the genitals and which became an object of fashion by around 1450 (although men had earlier discovered its practicality during combat).

What began as a modest accessory soon changed into an object of display, made of silk and decorated with ribbons and precious stones. Not infrequently they were enlarged with stuffing.

However, the fact remains that we've all grown up with the idea that there is something sexy about nudity, especially with the opposite sex. What might lead you to question this idea is the actual experience of social nudity. This experience can convince you—in a way that historical arguments probably cannot—that something you have been taught to believe from the time you were little simply is *not* true.

THE FEAR OF PUBLIC NUDITY

Most people who have never experienced social nudity either can't imagine what might happen if they were to take their clothes off—or else they *can* imagine, and don't like what they imagine. Rarely do expectations reflect the reality of what does happen when one goes naked in front of others for the first time.

The thought of men walking around with erections visible to everyone causes some of the embarrassment many people feel when they think of a nudist camp or nude beach.

That is because most people associate *nude* with *sexy*. The reason for the association is that usually the only time men and women have their clothes off in the presence of another person is in situations where there is the possibility of having sex. We have been conditioned to expect nudity and sex *always* go together.

Men say quite frankly that they fear they will have an erection. Women say they fear their bodies will not be considered attractive enough. (Both sexes also worry about being considered too fat.) There is another set of concerns that most people are not even aware of: men fear they will *not* have an erection; women fear their bodies will be considered *too* attractive.

What Men Fear

Most men express concern that the sight of all those bare breasts and bottoms at a nude beach or resort is bound to cause an erection. Emily encountered this argument from her gynecologist when he discovered she had acquired her all-over tan at Elysium:

> "What about the men? What about their erections?" he said to me, as though accusing me of being interested only in my own jollies, oblivious of the discomfort my and other women's nudity would cause men.
>
> "Well, what about their erections?" I countered. By this time I was used to questions about erections, and used to strong emotional reactions to my admission of indulging in social nudity.
>
> "It's not healthy for men to get so fired up, to get their sex organs engorged if there is no place around to get release. That's what causes prostatitis," he said, seeming indignant at my ignorance.
>
> "What's going to cause all this excitement?" I asked, knowing in advance what his answer would be.
>
> "Well, the sight of those women—their breasts and . . . and things." The learned doctor stuttered like a schoolboy trying to say unfamiliar words.
>
> "Really, now," I said (very condescendingly, I'll have to admit—I hadn't liked his implying that I was

both ignorant and uncaring), "you make your living looking at what are supposed to be the most sexually provocative parts of women. You do it all day long. What do you do about *your* erections? Do you have prostatitis?"

He shrugged his shoulders, smiled wanly and didn't answer, but his questioning took a different direction and was pursued with less of an air of moral indignation. He had suddenly realized he was himself proof that the sight of a naked woman or her sexual parts does not of itself, in all settings, produce an erection, sexual excitement, or even sexual interest.

What, in fact, *would* happen if a man developed an erection at a nude resort? Would everyone stare or point him out? Would women turn away? Would he be led off the grounds in disgrace? The answer is no on all counts. Probably no one would notice; if anyone did notice, there would be no fuss. Those used to group nudity tend to be pretty philosophical about bodily functions and are not likely to be any more upset by the swelling of a bit of erectile tissue than by the appearance of goose pimples.

It is not likely that a newcomer to a social nudity situation will have an erection. In the first place, a man is usually so nervous that he couldn't make it happen even if he wanted to. As every grown male knows, when he is nervous and anxious, it is extremely difficult to relax enough so that an erection can happen. One nude-resort owner we know is willing to bet a first-time visitor anywhere from five to one hundred dollars that he won't get an erection on his first visit. And though men have been taking him up on his bet for over twenty years, he has not lost once. This may be a bit of an overstatement because a relatively rare man will have an erection.

A nudist camp or nude beach does not provide the kind of environment that stimulates sexual arousal. Completely missing is the kind of sexual titillation present at a strip-tease or topless-bottomless show. The sight of sweaty people playing volleyball, sitting in the sun, or jogging, or children playing in the sand, are not sexually arousing sights for most persons.

Many men are also afraid that the sight of so many naked women will make them blasé, that later, at an appropriate time with a sex partner, they will *not* be able to have an erection. However, social nudity, rather than making a man impotent, is likely to have a positive influence on his sex life. Dr. William Hartman and Marilyn Fithian observed that the practice of social nudism often brought about an increase in the frequency of sexual intercourse, as well as an increase in overall sexual happiness.

In addition to concerns about erection, many men are self-conscious about the way their penises look. While most fear being considered too small, a few worry they are too large. These fears usually disappear when a man sees the sex organs of many other men—some of whom are sure to have larger penises and some smaller.

What Women Fear

A woman's primary worry about social nudity is how she will look naked, and this, of course, reflects the fact that women in our society have been educated to feel their major value lies in being attractive to men. Believing that the only way men will find them attractive is if they look beautiful, they spend considerable time and money on hairdos, make-up, and cosmetic surgery, as well as on bras, girdles, and clothes designed to conceal bodily "imperfections."

Every generation has had its ideal of female pulchritude, and those trying to copy the eighteen-inch waistline of Scarlett O'Hara's day could fake it with waist cinchers, padding, and binding. But today's woman, competing with the *Playboy* centerfold, believes that when naked, she is inadequate unless she looks youthful, unblemished, and well-proportioned. (She doesn't realize that even the Playmate of the Month requires a great deal of fussing with camera angles, lights, and even gravity to achieve that illusion of perfection.)

With such an impossible ideal to live up to, it's the rare woman who isn't unhappy about some aspect of her appearance. Usually it's her breasts, which seem to come in only two sizes—too large and too small. Or they sag. Or they are too far apart. Or the nipples aren't right. Women are also concerned with stretchmarks, fat hips, fat tummies, and fat thighs or else about being too skinny and/or masculine-looking.

A social nudity experience can introduce women to reality. As a thirty-five-year-old divorced mother of three exclaimed after her first visit to a nude beach, "It was so great! I didn't have to enter the bathing suit competition. Ordinarily my stomach hangs over my suit. It's not so obvious when I'm nude. Besides, the other women have stomachs too. Now I'm getting to accept the fact that I have a stomach, and it's okay."

Women have a second worry about social nudity—the fear that men will find them *too* sexually attractive, get aroused, and expect to have sex. Because a woman has been encouraged since birth to exhibit herself to males by wearing provocative or revealing clothing, it is no wonder she fears men will be sexually stimulated by the ultimate exhibit—her naked body.

There is another concern that a woman may not be consciously aware of: she may believe that being nude in front of a man she doesn't intend to have sex with is apt to make her a "tease," a woman who deliberately arouses desire she has no intention of satisfying. Some women fear rape—and even that they would deserve it—if they were to reveal their bodies.

But you aren't a tease and you won't be raped. The sight of female breasts and genitalia does not usually stimulate a desire for sex unless these body parts are displayed in a sexually provocative way or the *intent* is to have sex. After all, the sight of the naked primitives in *National Geographic* or of a mother nursing her baby does not usually cause sexual arousal in men.

Getting used to being looked at—so used to it that it doesn't worry her—is a good experience for a woman. It is a relief to discover that no matter how unattractive a woman believes her body to be, no one will turn away in disgust or shun her. Nor will she be sexually molested. A woman's thoughts and behavior may change as a result of the discovery that the appearance of her body will neither send men away nor turn them into rapists.

Fear of Fat

Almost everybody in this country considers themselves overweight, judging from the most common excuse given for not trying social nudity: "I'd do it if I were ten pounds lighter." Whether you are overweight or whether you imagine you are, your confidence and functioning depend on the way you feel about your body. If you fear others in a social nudity situation will find your body repulsive and reject you as a result, that fear is real and a part of you, and it affects you whether you have your clothes on or off. If such a fear keeps you from taking off your clothes in public, you are missing a great opportunity. Many "fatties" have learned to love their own fat and thus to love themselves *as they are* because of the very casual acceptance of their bodies by others in nude workshops, at nude beaches, nude resorts, etc.

Countless times we have seen the apprehension on the faces of overweight people trying social nudity for the first time change to delight as they realize no one notices their fat or if they notice, they simply don't care. We've interviewed many fat people in social nudity settings and discovered that they have become more accepting and tolerant of their own bodies as a result of finding out others not only accept them but even like them *as is*. Psychotherapists have told us of patients—some grossly fat—whose self-esteem increased so much after a social nudity experience that it led to improvements in their relationships—and, in some cases, *to a subsequent loss of weight*. (The theory is that you have to psychologically accept your body before you can change it.)

If overweight is the only reason you are fearful of trying a social nudity experience, consider these reasons why you shouldn't wait until that magic day when you lose ten or twenty or even a hundred pounds. In the first place, one-fourth of all Americans are overweight, and it's no wonder. Present day social life usually revolves around eating and drinking; the quick-foods so many of us rely on are usually heavy in carbohydrates, fat, and calories. In addition, since childhood most of us have been taught to satisfy our emotional needs orally—with a coke, a cookie, a sandwich. The tensions of modern life make many of us turn more and more to sources of oral gratification. Until our entire society makes some significant changes in the way we live and eat, many of us will always have to struggle with weight problems.

In the second place, though many of us are overweight and though we are encouraged to overeat, we are prejudiced against fat at least partly because of society's rigid sex stereotypes and tendency to devaluate what is feminine. Slim hips, slender thighs, and a flat tummy are desired by men and women alike. Yet these desires are more difficult for women to realize since they tend to have more fleshy stomachs, buttocks, and thighs than males.

Our society sees slender as good and fat as bad. As a result, both men and women can be victims of their own unrealistic cultural expectations and can fail to see beauty in the bodies of others who don't fit the masculine or feminine ideal.

A man with a little extra fat on his stomach or chest or buttocks, or one who has a body build that tends more to round and soft than angular and muscular, may worry about not looking "masculine." And indeed those who look at him may judge him as not being masculine, unaware that it is behavior that counts, not pounds or inches. A woman who weighs 110 pounds may make herself miserable trying to do something about the "fat" thighs that are a mark of her genetic heritage and which were admired in past centuries and glorified by painters such as Rubens, Rembrandt, and Botticelli.

SOCIAL NUDITY IS FOR EVERYONE

Some elderly people attain a simple dignity unclothed that they do not have when dressed in the drab manner many of them adopt. Some teenagers, obscured when dressed in the latest fads, blossom into exuberant and graceful sprites undressed. Body features that may be diverting when a person is dressed—such as a belly that bulges over a tight belt, wooly chest hair that protrudes from the neck of a sport shirt, or legs that look spindly in a short skirt, seem attractive and in harmony when seen as integral parts of an entire body.

People who feel self-conscious about birthmarks, scars, stretchmarks, wrinkled or sagging skin, varicose veins, or a missing breast or limb can benefit from social nudity. It can help such people realize that a deviation from society's norms is seldom the primary cause of a person's problems or unhappiness and never the only cause.

We've talked a lot about fears of social nudity and you've probably identified several as your own. It might be helpful to take another look at the questionnaires at the end of chapters one and two to see if you can get some clues as to what aspect of body prejudice might be making you reluctant to try social nudity.

Taking Off Your Clothes for the First Time

The most common reaction of people after their first social nudity experience is one of surprise: at how easy it was, at how their uncomfortable feelings quickly disappeared, and that nothing bad happened. In fact, most people who can recall their first nude experience agree with Alex Comfort that

> "the ingrained taboo of genital concealment, which makes most of us self-conscious at the idea of undressing before strangers, has a lifetime of about fifteen minutes in a community that ignores it."

Interestingly enough, it is probably *easier* to get over your fears and self-consciousness in a community of strangers than it is with your friends. With strangers you will never have to see again, it is easier to risk looking foolish or exposing parts of yourself you think ugly or unacceptable.

For most people the safest and most appropriate places to begin participatory nudity are communities of strangers where going bare is taken for granted, such as nude workshops, beaches, resorts, and travel tours. We will describe each of these in the next two chapters.

Looking at Others

Just as people have fears about being looked at in a group nudity situation, they have fears about looking at others. They are reluctant to be caught staring, and don't realize that looking and staring are two different things. Staring is offensive to other people. It dehumanizes them and makes them feel like objects. On the other hand, looking at a person acknowledges that he is a complete human being—not just a collection of anatomical parts. To look instead of stare, soften your gaze and look at that person as though gently stroking him or her with your eyes.

1. Look at foreheads, eyes, noses, cheeks, mouths, chins, ears, and hair. *Describe* them to yourself ("Her forehead is very high; his has pimples on it; that one has bushy eyebrows"). After describing, take time to *evaluate* what you see ("This one has pretty skin; that one has a friendly mouth; the other one has bedroom eyes"). After evaluating, take time to become aware of how what you perceive makes you *feel* ("his unsmiling face makes me want to turn away; his handsome, dimpled chin makes me feel inferior because I have a receding jaw").

2. Next look at necks, arms, and hands. Become aware of a person's movements as well as the parts of his body. Describe these movements to yourself ("She flutters her hands a lot"). Judge the movements ("It's fun to watch her hands, especially her thumbs"). Become aware of underlying assumptions you make ("I wouldn't want her to dry my dishes—she is apt to let them slip through her fingers").

3. Examine different parts of the upper torso, then the pubic area and hips, then the legs and feet.

4. If some person or some particular part of a person's anatomy intrigues you, examine it until you've seen as much as you want. (The attributes you notice most of all, particularly those that please you or bother you, may indicate what concerns you. For example, if you notice a lot of very dark, bushy pubic hair, it may be that you are concerned that your own is too dark and too bushy or too pale and sparse.) Do your looking in short periods. Look away frequently. Look at other people or read a book or whatever. It is possible to get your fill of looking—to enjoy and to learn a lot about other people and about yourself—without making anyone feel you are spying.

5. When you have gotten your fill of examining chest hair, nipples, belly buttons, or whatever, start looking at parts of people's bodies and attributing personality characteristics to the person on the basis of what you see. We frequently look at people's faces and judge them as flirty, arrogant, wholesome, business-like, etc. Try doing the same with other aspects of the body. Naturally, the characteristics you attribute to a person on the basis of bodily appearance may not prove valid, but the exercise will help make you aware of your assumptions and more observant.

Chapter 11
Accepting Yourself in a Brave Nude World

I exist as I am, that is enough.

> Walt Whitman,
> *Song of Myself*

Body liberation workshops, which are off-shoots of body liberation therapy, provide the kind of structured setting that helps a person examine, and possibly discard, some of his body prejudice—the attitudes and perceptions that may have given him a lifetime of negative body feelings. Workshops focus on introducing new concepts and educational exercises, and have particular goals, such as sexual enhancement, improvement of body image, and improvement of man-woman relationships. Unlike in therapy, the leader does not probe deep into the psyche of the participants.

To give you an idea of what it is like to go nude in public for the first time in an educational setting, let us describe one of a variety of Emily Coleman's clothing-optional workshops.

EMILY'S WORKSHOP

Emily is not a therapist and does not practice therapy. She is an educator who has probably taught more classes in which nudity was an integral part than any other educator. Designed to introduce people to their own bodies and to the bodies of others, and to promote bodily acceptance in a very short time, this workshop is called "Brave Nude World." Groups vary in size from six to ninety and workshops have had a wide range of settings, from a college conference center to a church camp grounds to a baronial mansion in England. "Brave Nude World" is her shortest workshop, lasting three hours. It includes a brief lecture, considerable group discussion, a demonstration, and a series of three exercises, each of which helps participants confront a body taboo in a safely structured atmosphere.

The purpose of the workshop is threefold:

1. To encourage realistic body perception—to help each participant get a sense of his body as it truly *is*, rather than as he would like it to be or fears it is.

2. To increase a participant's awareness of the effect the appearance of his body has on others.

3. To help him understand and eliminate some unreal fears of looking at the bodies of others, of being seen, of touching and being touched—fears which underlie behavior and interfere with the enjoyable, effective use of his body even when clothed.

The particular workshop we will describe was held in Santa Barbara, California, and was part of a five-day conference on male-female relationships. To convey the three hours most directly and vividly, we will describe them from two points of view, first that of Betty Edwards as she experienced this type of workshop for the first time, then that of Emily as leader.

Betty tells what she felt and saw as the participants gathered in a large carpeted room shortly before the workshop was scheduled to start.

Betty's View

I feel like a pioneer. Attending a nude workshop for the purpose of learning about my own body is hardly an everyday occurrence in my life. I also feel like a voyeur, since as Emily's writing collaborator I am to observe the other participants. I look calmer than I feel. I quiet the butterflies in my stomach by walking around doing interviews, submerging my own qualms by listening to those of forty men and women of all ages, sizes, shapes, and occupations.

"I'm a little nervous at the idea of being shut up in this bright room, taking off my clothes, and being next to so many nude bodies," one gray-haired woman says plaintively. "I've been in massage workshops outdoors where we were all nude, but somehow nudity seems more natural in the open air."

She takes a deep breath and sits down, apparently reassured when someone tells her that nudity is completely optional. Not only is it acceptable to remain dressed, but Emily will give reinforcement to those who do *not* choose to undress.

"I haven't decided whether or not I'll take my clothes off," says a red-bearded man, his arms folded tightly over a tie-dye T-shirt. "I'm going to wait and see what happens."

"Not me," responds a young woman with oversized dark glasses. "I didn't come this far and go to this much trouble to stay dressed."

"Now, remember," an anxious wife reminds her husband, "you promised you wouldn't pressure me to get undressed, if I agreed to come with you to this."

My fellow participants are not avant-garde sophisticates seeking sex thrills. They are ordinary people with all the ordinary hangups about their bodies. But they are willing to explore a taboo area, and for most, this will be their first nude experience.

We nervously mill around the room waiting for Emily to begin. I am regretting the extra goodies I've eaten over the last six months, which contributed to a roll of fat around my waist. I am not alone in feeling that my body won't measure up.

A pale-skinned high school teacher in a Hawaiian muumuu expresses a common insecurity among women: "I've never been in a situation where people were nude, except individually, and I feel all the imperfections in myself. After all, I'm fifty-two years old and overweight. If I were twenty-four and slim, maybe I wouldn't mind."

Others worry about being found out by friends, employers, or relatives. Everyone is fully clothed, but there is a general scurrying to be out of camera range when a newspaper photographer reporting on the conference enters the room. People relax only after he assures them he is just shooting Emily and the back of people's heads.

"My god," gasps a young man, "my boss would flip if he saw a picture of me here."

"I don't have a boss to worry about," says an olive-skinned young woman, "but my mother would be horrified. She'd think we were screwing in every corner."

I wander through the crowd, listening to pieces of conversation.

"I hate my body and want to find out why my husband likes it."

"My therapist thought this workshop would be good for me."

"If the PTA ladies could only see me now."

"I wouldn't be here today if it weren't for Emily. I'm scared as hell, but I've been in some of her other workshops and I trust her and know it will be okay."

After a while we sit down on the carpet and wait apprehensively for Emily to begin.

Emily's View

Most of the people who come to my workshops are motivated by one or more of the following:

1. Most want new experiences to stimulate personal and social growth.

2. Some want to improve their sex lives and believe that through social nudity they can learn to feel more relaxed in future sexual activities.

3. Some have bad feelings about their bodies as a whole or about particular parts. Some have bad feelings about the aging process.

4. Some want to get over hangups about taking off their clothes. They want to stop associating nudity with silliness or sin.

5. Some are here as a result of pressure from a spouse or lover.

6. Some have been sent by their therapists.

Whatever their motivations, persons vary tremendously in their readiness to shed fears, to talk about feelings, and to trust. People must trust before they dare to try a new and frightening experience, and I have to work very hard at first to help them build trust in me. I do so by sharing my own emotions and experiences.

As I talk, the men and women in the room begin to relax. I had once experienced all of their fears. Soon it is apparent to them that I am not a kook but a motherly person who went through a lot to become comfortable with her own body.

Before long, people excitedly, shyly, or nervously begin to tell about their own previous nude experiences, their worries (shared by most other participants), and their hopes of what this body liberation workshop will do for them. I make certain that each person who speaks gets approval from me, no matter what his feelings, opinions, or experiences. It takes a lot of courage to share such intimate revelations with strangers.

I assure participants that they are not going to be asked to do anything they don't want to do and that nothing will be done to them against their will. The people who come to my workshops seem especially conscientious and cooperative, and I have never experienced or witnessed any objectionable behavior from any of them.

I never know just how long I will talk about fears with a new group. The warm-up period is important, for it sets a mood for what follows. Though it usually lasts for ten to thirty minutes, I don't watch the clock, but simply talk until I sense that a certain level of trust has developed. Then I move to the next stage, inviting participants to join me in a new learning experience—the first of the three exercises.

Students are asked to close their eyes and, with all their clothes on and under my guidance, to carefully and sensitively explore their own bodies. I caution them not to do anything they do not want to do, but at the same time I encourage them to push themselves a little bit. I tell them they are free to not participate at all, to hold back and get a late start, or to stop whenever they become too uncomfortable. Each person has his own pace.

Betty's View

Like a tour director, Emily confidently guides our exploration of strange terrain. I close my eyes as she suggests. I've never touched and felt my body in quite this way before and doubt if the others have either.

"Put your hands to your head and touch your hair," she directs. "Notice its texture and softness. How does it feel to your hands? How do your hands feel to your hair?"

I am surprised to discover it is a pleasurable sensation to feel my own hair—surprised to discover there are two of me, one who feels the hair and one whose hair is felt.

I cannot resist peeking at the others, and watch as forty pairs of hands scratch, pull, and caress forty heads of hair. Many persons are smiling, caught up in rediscovering themselves.

"Explore your face," Emily continues, "and feel your skin temperature. How does your face feel to your hands? How do your hands feel to your face?"

We slowly explore all parts of our bodies—neck, shoulders, arms, chest, stomach, buttocks, genitals, legs, feet—asking ourselves how we feel about each part.

Then Emily asks us to touch the part we like the best and the part we like the least. My breasts are my favorite part and my stomach the part I like the least. My breasts feel good because they are big, round, and soft. Yet so is my stomach. Why can't I enjoy both? Obviously I've gotten the idea that stomachs must be flat.

I speak up and tell the others what I am thinking, though I worry they will put me down for admitting I have a big stomach. Instead they applaud. Several men say they like the feel of soft bellies on women. Several other women talk about their feelings toward their big bellies.

A trim woman of forty-five disagrees that soft bellies are preferable. She asks us to feel her flat stomach, the result of countless hours of exercise. Some of us feel and admire her stomach. Suddenly I see that there are no absolutes. I sit back, hands on my belly, enjoying the softness.

A retired Air Force officer and pilot confesses he senses a loss of vigor when he feels his body, particularly his arms. To the group he appears to be a powerful man, but much of his self-image has been based on his strength which has lessened in recent years. It occurs to him that he can no longer rely on his muscles to attract women.

One woman tells him that she is attracted to him not because of his build but because he is an interesting, sensitive person. The man begins to see that maybe his pride in his physique kept him from being aware of his other desirable qualities. Sometimes the loss of one kind of strength can be the beginning of another.

Emily's View

The time of the big decision has arrived—to strip or not to strip, that is the question. Whenever I ask my students to do anything I consider difficult, I demonstrate by doing it first. When trying something new and difficult, everyone needs someone to jump the hurdles first and call back, "Come on, you can do it." Though it has been many years since I first participated in group nudity, I dread this moment. It is not easy to stand up and take off your clothes while a whole roomful of properly attired people sit back and watch your every move and expression. Yet I also look forward to the experience, seeing it as the bullfighter's moment of truth.

Always I dress carefully for the occasion—no undergarments to fumble with, only a long dress with a minimum of buttons, a dress that I can slip off easily, up and over my head.

I sweat profusely as the time approaches. I think of past moments of shame and embarrassment, of risk and triumph. An odd assortment of memories are triggered: *The time I was seven and had a cold, and while my mother was rubbing my bare chest with camphorated oil, I—horrors—saw a neighbor boy peeking at me through the window. The time I was ten and the nuns wouldn't let me perform my first piano recital because my new dress didn't cover my elbows—anger, disappointment, relief. The time I was thirteen and had to pull down my underpants to let the doctor give me a shot.* My thoughts turn from the past to the present, from embarrassment to a feeling of pride.

Betty's View

Smiling, calm, Emily removes her long black dress, and suddenly is standing before us completely nude. It could have been a vulgar moment, like a stripper taking off a G-string; it could have been a clinical moment, like a cadaver unveiled for anatomy students; it could have been an uncomfortable moment, like being forced to witness someone's public humiliation. But it is an inspiring moment.

Emily then touches her own body from head to toe, telling how she feels about each area. She tells us she likes her breasts and small waistline, has been convinced by admirers she has a remarkable fanny, thinks her face is not pretty, and wishes that her thighs and stomach weren't so fat.

Emily's View

After I have taken off my clothing, touched and talked about my body, allowed others to touch me, I state the instructions for the second exercise:

1. I tell the participants to form groups of four, five, or six.

2. I instruct each person to decide for himself how many—if any—of his garments he wants to remove, and then to remove them.

3. I direct each person, one at a time, without questions or comments from others, to stand and touch the parts of his body, from head to toe. As he does so, he is to tell the other group members what he likes and dislikes about his body.

4. When he has finished, I ask the group members to tell him what about his body they liked and didn't like.

When everyone has had a turn, the third exercise begins:

1. Participants may offer to let others touch their body parts or ask others if they can touch particular parts of their bodies. Anyone may refuse any request or put a stop to any touching.

2. I ask people to become aware of thoughts or feelings that make them do what they do.

Betty's View

Six of us are sitting in a small circle, with instructions to share intimate feelings about our bodies—feelings we have kept hidden even from ourselves. There is Marcia, a housewife of thirty who is extremely obese; Jack, a powerfully built construction worker; Peggy, a beautiful young college student; Ernie, an industrial psychologist in his forties; Bill, a fifty-five-year-old businessman; and me, conscious of every extra pound, wrinkle, and year on my body. One by one, we stand up before our small group and point out everything we like and don't like about our bodies. For instance, Peggy, the college student, says:

> I'm learning to like my hair. Sometimes I worry about my skin because it breaks out... and I pluck my eyebrows instead of just accepting them the way they are.... Some people tease me about my nose, but I think it is okay. I like my body. I like my coloring when I am tan. I worry about my shoulders because one is higher than the other. Also this breast is bigger than this one, but I like how my breasts feel.... I can go without a bra. I am of medium size, so I never worry about being too small or too big. I like my stomach although it is a little bit round. I used to make it very flat but I've been learning it is better to have it softer. I guess I never thought about my pubic hair but I've been getting compliments. I like how my legs look when they are tan—and the shape of them. But sometimes I think they are too fat.

We tell her what we like about her body. Ernie likes her hair; Marcia likes her muscletone; and I like her small ribcage.

We have trouble giving negative feedback. Bill thinks that if we feel something negative, we should be able to say it rather than holding back. Jack thinks that if someone has strong feelings, he should express them. Marcia finds it hard to give feedback that is not complimentary. As an expert on criticizing myself, the one thing I don't need is people telling me what they don't like.

When it is my turn to stand up in front of the group, my negative feelings about my body come out. Nothing in my life has prepared me for the terror of that moment. I stand totally naked and unprotected before strangers, revealing myself both physically and emotionally.

I run my hands over my face feeling the wrinkles, sags, and double chin. It's a jolt to acknowledge that I am a middle-aged woman, not the young girl I sometimes feel inside. I touch the soft undersides of my upper arms and the excess flesh on my waistline, and I realize I am somewhat more than voluptuous—I am downright overweight. The stretchmarks on my belly tell me I'm no longer brand new. I bear the marks of living.

My group members show no contempt for my flaws. They take me as I am. And because they like me, I'm able to take a second look at myself.

I feel my shoulders, back, arms, and legs. They are strong. I begin to see myself—really see myself—for what I am. I am flawed and perfect, powerful and needy, young and old—and alive.

The third exercise calls for us, one at a time, to ask other group members if they would like to touch any parts of our bodies—realizing we and they can say yes or no. Touching Marcia, I realize that—despite all of society's conditioning—fat is not disgusting but warm and soft. Touching Jack, I realize that I can enjoy the different feel of a man's body without wanting to have sex. Touching Peggy, I realize that stroking a beautiful woman's smooth skin can be a sensual, rather than a sexual, experience.

Suddenly the rest of us are denied the experience of being touched because Emily decrees (by ringing a little bell) that the exercise is over. We protest. We want to stay together and continue this experience a little longer. We don't want to let go of it and return to the world where people don't touch each other and don't accept each other.

Emily's View

I set time limits for all activities in which the students work in small groups, independent of me. The time limit adds a feeling of safety, making it easier for participants who may be uncomfortable or who may have revealed more than they intended to. They know a graceful exit will be possible.

Often I am asked why I suggest that people tell each other what they don't like about each other's bodies, instead of just what they do like.

There are four reasons:

1. People appreciate, want, need, and feel more comfortable with honesty. You wouldn't learn or grow much as a

member of a compliment club. You can't trust the compliments of a person who won't also tell you what he doesn't like.

2. People need practice at learning to express dislikes as personal reactions rather than definitive judgments. This takes the sting out of negative feedback.

3. When dislikes are freely expressed—as personal reactions—it becomes apparent that frequently what one person dislikes, another likes. There is nothing about a person's body that is repulsive to everybody. Likes depend upon experiences and expectations. What we see reminds us of people and incidents out of the past, and of our hopes for the future, and we like or dislike accordingly.

4. Most people fool themselves about the appearance of their bodies. Self-deception interferes with personal development and happiness, with the ability to work with *what is* in order to create *what can be*.

I end the workshop with group participation in a particularly tender method of touching (the Von Newman massage, described in Chapter 14). Touching exercises done in the nude help people learn to experience each other through their *senses*, and in a natural way, instead of only through their *minds*.

Carefully structured exercises, such as the ones in my workshop, done by willing participants in an atmosphere of trust, can help people get over many of the fears that accompany touching and being touched.

Betty's View

After the Von Newman massage, we talk about the morning's experiences. Looking at the assortment of bodies, a woman says, "When you were dressed you all looked alike, but now you are all individuals and beautiful."

"This is so great," someone else says, "but, Emily, you talked for so long, using time we could have spent enjoying being undressed together."

Emily laughs and points out that the kind of talking done was necessary as a starter. We wouldn't have enjoyed our nude experiences so much without all that talking. She looks around at the naked people sprawled contentedly on beach towels and mats and teasingly asks, "I don't suppose you want to break for lunch. Shall I have it sent in?"

"Yes," we eagerly answer. We are reluctant to end an experience that has been unlike any other. Emily permits us to go "overtime" for a few minutes and talk more about the insights we have gained.

One man is delighted by the discovery that his hairiness did not turn people off, while another man is relieved that his relatively hairless body is also acceptable.

A petite redhead is chuckling because during the workshop someone told her that her body, which is covered with small black moles, looks like a chocolate chip cookie.

Another young woman giggles and remarks, "I never knew penises could look so different."

I, too, have made an important discovery. With clothes off, men no longer seem smarter and more powerful than women. Men are people—vulnerable like me.

Emily has not just been indulging us by letting us express our feelings and new thoughts. Being able to articulate our feelings and insights helps us internalize our new learning so we will be able to use it in the future. Although I think the others, like me, have been changed in many important ways, most of us can't yet define clearly what has happened to us.

Most of us are ready for other social nudity experiences.

POSTSCRIPT

Although there are no other workshops exactly like "Brave Nude World" (one that facilitates in a very short time the removal of clothing, the touching of nude bodies, and the acquisition of new feelings and attitudes) there are many other excellent body-liberating workshops focusing on such areas as body image, sensory awareness, massage, and sexual enhancement. Many permit nudity. Such workshops are offered in day-long, weekend, or weekly courses at growth centers, holistic health centers, women's centers, universities, and even churches.

Chapter 12
Nude Beaches, Resorts, and Travel Tours

> A free beach is a place where people find a liberation from the trappings of civilization and share the common denominator of being their simplest selves. Their code is to let one be as long as there is no personal intrusion. It's so simple that many folks find it a wonder that *all* the beaches and river banks of America are not already free.
>
> Leon Elder,
> *Free Beaches: A Phenomenon
> of the California Coast*

While almost every other place for socializing has a tradition and structure geared to the wearing of clothing, nude beaches and resorts are special places with a tradition and structure that facilitate a newcomer's acceptance of his own and others' nudity.

In these special environments, although you will not have a skilled leader to help you become aware of and deal with your feelings, you can achieve many body liberation benefits. To get the most out of this new experience, you have to put yourself in charge. We can only give you guidelines, try to allay your fears, and let you know what to expect.

First of all, try not to be concerned with how others may be seeing you. Pay attention to your own experiences and sensations—the feeling of sun and sand, for example—rather than to how others may be experiencing you.

Nude beaches, nudist resorts (the new term for nudist camps), and nude tours provide good ways of experiencing going bare in public for the first time.

In fact, these places have made it easier for some families to make the transition from being an always-clothed family to being a sometimes-unclothed family. Going together as a family to a nude beach or camp filled with hundreds of people of all ages, sizes, and shapes can help lessen any embarrassment that might arise when parents and children take off their clothes together for the first time. The shock or embarrassment simply can't be too great or last too long when you are surrounded by so many others to whom nudity is casual and matter-of-fact. Both children and parents tend to get caught up in the panorama of life they see around them—pregnant mothers, tiny babies, older children, teenagers, adults, and oldsters. They can see that bodies are ever-changing and their own nudity, too, becomes a natural part of life.

Before taking your children to a nudist camp or nude beach, we advise:

1. Be cautious about the nude beach to which you take your children. Go by yourselves once to make sure the beach you've chosen is a family-oriented one.

2. A nudist camp is more predictable than a nude beach in terms of what you can expect. Most of them will have activities for young people.

CLOTHING-OPTIONAL BEACHES

Nude, free, or clothing-optional beaches—the terms are interchangeable—are places where swimsuits are optional. Most such beaches are found in California, Oregon, New York, Massachusetts, and Florida, but there are also many inland lakes and streams throughout the country where public nude swimming and sunbathing takes place.

A major advantage in going to a nude beach for your first experience is that it is perfectly all right to wear your swimsuit until you feel comfortable taking it off. As a result you can give the experience a try, knowing you won't look ridiculous or out of place if you don't undress. People are free to wear what they feel like wearing. A man may wear a T-shirt and jeans because he is modest or because he has a sunburn and needs to keep covered. A woman may wear just her bathing suit bottom because she is menstruating or because she is shy about exposing that part of her body. A member of either sex may go nude most of the time but put on a sweater if the day is windy or cold. Probably no one will pay any attention to you no matter what you wear (unless it is something decidedly out of place for any beach, such as a business suit).

Despite the fact that the legal status of nude beaches has not yet been clearly defined throughout the nation (we'll discuss this further in Chapter 15), there are beaches where it is now okay to go nude. Some public beaches (Black's Beach in San Diego, California, for example) are legal. Some beaches (such as the Red, White, and Blue Beach in Santa Cruz, California) are privately owned and charge admission. At some public beaches where nudity is not officially legal, the authorities unofficially tolerate it because of long-established local custom, relatively small numbers of nude bathers, or lack of media publicity.

Clothing-optional beaches vary as much as do traditional beaches (called "textile beaches" by free-beachers), not just in the quality of surf and sand but in the personality and behavior of the people who go there. Some (i.e., the Red, White, and Blue Beach) are particularly safe for newcomers because the owners enforce their own rules and regulations. Other beaches (like Brooks Beach in Venice, California, before nudity was banned in 1974) have a more counter-culture atmosphere with happy hippies, gorgeous gays, and a number of gawkers. Pirate's Cove, a privately owned beach in Southern California (where nudity is unofficially permitted) has a family atmosphere, with adults and children unself-consciously enjoying sun and surf.

In fact, it was an experience at Pirate's Cove that got one family started on enjoying all the pleasure and benefits of family nudity. Norman was talked into going to a free beach by his wife, Jean, who wanted to experience group nudity in an outdoor environment. After three or four times, he became a convert to the pleasures and benefits of nudity—so much so that he wanted to take their twelve-year-old daughter, Sandy. Now it was Jean's turn to be reluctant; she was worried about the effect the experience would have on Sandy, who had never seen them nude.

Norman felt that Sandy would not be bothered if they introduced her to nudity in a way that seemed natural and ordinary. So they told Sandy they were all going to the beach and added, "But we think you'll be surprised." (We believe it is best to advise children if you plan to take them into a nude situation, but in this case the surprise turned out well.) Norman tells what happened at the beach:

> Sandy was very nonchalant. She was either able to hide her feelings or was not very affected by the surprise. It was quite hot, and after a while she asked our permission to take off her suit. We took off our suits while she was in swimming and when she got back to the blanket she was very pleased that we had joined her and the rest of the crowd in going *au naturel.* When we got home, we all talked for hours about the experience and how we felt about it. Sandy thought it was a nice surprise and wondered why we hadn't taken her sooner.

A natural atmosphere is a characteristic of most nude beaches. They simply bring into the daylight and public view something most of us have done at one time or another—skinny dip. The freedom of a nude beach combined with the beauty of the water, sun, sand and bodies makes most people feel carefree, joyous, and sometimes childlike. A middle-aged friend of ours said:

> I felt like I was a little naked two-year-old playing in the surf. I romped, the waves knocked me down, I laughed, I splashed. I haven't had so much fun in years. Then as I was walking out of the water I put my hands on my breasts and realized I had no top on. For a minute I panicked—like in the dream where you realize you are naked in a public place and everyone is staring. Then I remembered where I was and that it was okay.

In addition to the sheer pleasure nude bathing and sunning bring, there are practical advantages. Bathing suits are expensive (in 1974 American women spent over $100 million on bathing suits) and often uncomfortable. As Rod Swenson wrote in *Penthouse* magazine, a bathing suit is "clammy; it gets full of sand when you're on the beach; it leaves suntan lines on your body; and it's still dripping wet when the rest of you is already dry."

Many people stay away from nude beaches because they worry about "voyeurs"—fully dressed men who wander around the beach staring at people. (Interestingly, women are never considered voyeurs even if they wander around staring.) Since there is no law against looking and since lawmakers cannot decide when looking ceases to be friendly and becomes objectionable, you may be looked at. Actually, it can be a beneficial experience for you to learn to remain unruffled when others look at you undressed. And your being tolerant of clothed sightseers can be therapeutic to them. Cec Cinder, member of the Board of Directors of *Beachfront USA*, says:

> Nude people are "teachers" in some respects for voyeurs. Chances are the person who is wandering through the crowd fully dressed and seeming to stare may be frightened, shy, or curious about viewing the human body—a body he has been taught to think of as base or wicked. Let him look! The experience will be an educational one for him and next week he may be back, but you won't recognize him because he is likely to be sitting next to you on the sand, nude, enjoying the sun.

In any event, at a nude beach people act pretty much the way they do at a traditional beach. Anyone drinking too much, making suggestive remarks, or having sex would be as out of place there as he would be at any public place.

NUDE RESORTS

Nudist resorts (or camps) are privately owned clubs supported by the yearly fees of the members (usually $20 to $150) or the daily fees of visitors ($1 to $7). Some are membership cooperatives (such as Glen Eden in California, owned and run by the members) and are difficult to visit without prior arrangements, but most resorts permit non-members to enter upon payment of a fee at the gate. Except for a few Southern states, nudist resorts are found all over the country, and their facilities, such as swimming pools and snack bars, must meet state health standards just as those of any other club or restaurant must.

However, as private clubs, nudist resorts exercise control over who gets in and who doesn't. The nudist members represent a rather conservative cross-section of American life. Most are married, with families, and above average in education and income. The majority of the men are professional or skilled workers and the majority of the women are housewives. However, unmarried couples and singles often are allowed membership.

You are almost certain to be admitted to a nudist resort if you are white, middle-class looking, and bring your family, spouse, or a companion of the opposite sex. Perhaps because of fears that blacks and whites might mingle sexually, nudist camps have tended to discriminate against blacks. Although some camps in the South still maintain a white-only policy, most nudist resorts are becoming less prejudiced.

Single women have no difficulty in getting admitted to any camp. In fact, camps encourage them to visit. On the other hand, a single man is likely to have trouble getting into a camp as a member or for a one-day visit; one California camp charges single males a fee of twenty dollars for a single visit. This reflects the fact that more single men than women are interested in going to nudist resorts, and owners fear that disproportionate numbers of lone men would drive away single women and families.

There is a reason nudist camps have been interested in maintaining their family oriented "image." With the founding of official "nudism" in this country in 1929, nudists became viewed with suspicion by the non-nudist majority who considered the camps sinful "dens of iniquity." Newspapers tended to distort any incident (such as a messy divorce) in which a nudist was involved—blaming all problems on nudism—and zealous public officials were always looking for any excuse to close the camps down. In reaction, nudists themselves set standards that would be beyond reproach. The traditional nudists all but denied the existence of human sexuality. In their zeal to proclaim the wholesomeness and naturalness of the human body and to break down the automatic connection in most people's minds between nudity and sex, the nudists went so far as to act as though they never had sexual feelings—ever—as a result of viewing the naked body of a fellow camp-member.

Thus nudist camps developed rules of conduct which today make them safe and predictable places to take children—and the kids will generally find plenty of playmates. The camps belonging to the largest and most powerful nationwide nudist organization, the American Sunbathing Association (with over one hundred member-camps), follow these guidelines:

1. *No unnecessary body contact.* Once interpreted so strictly that a man could not hold his own daughter on his lap, this rule has been relaxed considerably. Today, hand-holding or an affectionate arm around the shoulders is not apt to be noticed, though prolonged touching or massaging of the body may draw a gentle reprimand. Overt sexual behavior definitely will get you thrown out.

2. *No photography without permission.* At most camps photography is permitted, but only with the permission of the management and the person being photographed. This is both common courtesy and a custom to protect the anonymity of nudists.

3. *Alcohol must be used with moderation.* Originally, ASA camps permitted no alcohol at all, partly because nudists were interested in healthful living and partly to protect their family oriented image. Today, member camps of the ASA can make their own decision about alcohol, and most permit it, but drunkenness is not tolerated.

4. *One partner in a marriage cannot obtain membership without the other.* This rule is relaxed if a spouse is disabled or ill, or if there's been a legal separation. Even then, the spouse must provide notarized permission.

One point to consider before visiting any nudist resort is that they are *not* clothing-optional. While some camps allow females to visit a few times without undressing, the general rule is that you *must* go nude at a nude resort—unless you are dancing. (Nude dancing is not usually permitted, probably because of sexual fears.) However, nudists, like the rest of us, don't like to freeze, and it is permissible to wear clothing during cold weather and at night when it gets chilly.

While the existence of some rules make sense, remnants of a puritanical tradition linger in a few camps in the form of certain "thou shalt nots" that seem a bit difficult to interpret, much less enforce: "Please avoid offending anyone or you may be asked to leave," "Do not gossip or speak unkindly of any person," "Save your smutty jokes for workday pals," and "Filthy and vulgar talk around children and visitors not tolerated." At camps with rules such as these you might think twice about giving your girlfriend a massage with baby oil or about having a frank talk about sex.

The trend today is definitely toward a more permissive atmosphere at nudist camps. Many of them are billing themselves as nudist "resorts" in hopes of attracting the vacation dollars of non-nudist tourists.

You can find a variety of facilities and activities at most nudist resorts. Almost every camp will have a pool, lake, or river for swimming, and most have volleyball courts. Other attractions include art classes, tennis courts, shuffleboard courts, hiking trails, and clubhouses for meetings and dances. Almost all have some kind of overnight accommodations. While a few have luxurious rooms, most have only rustic cabins or permanent trailers for rent, or else they have facilities for trailers, camping spaces, or simply a place to put sleeping bags. You can buy food at most camps, and eating facilities range from snack bars to elaborate restaurants.

Nudist resorts sometimes hold contests to lure customers. Nude beauty pageants are always a big draw. One of the best-known is the Miss Nude World contest, held at the Four Seasons Nature Park in Ontario, Canada, to which various camps send candidates. There are also contests to select Ms. All-Bare America, Miss Nude Chubby, and Mr. Nude U.S.A., and there is even a Nudist Olympics.

Though you may believe that you just couldn't go to a nudist resort—that you'd never be able to shed your inhibitions and your clothes in front of strangers—your reaction might be like that of Sally, a young mother of two: "I'm claiming myself back. This is really me, the way I feel here.

To be this free and casual and open—running around and playing with my kids—that feels like the real Sally. I have hidden her, not only behind my clothes but also behind should and should-not, don't-do-this and don't-do-that. I like this Sally."

NUDE TRAVEL TOURS

One sign of the popularity of body liberation is the growth in travel tours to nude beaches and resorts in foreign countries. Here are a few of the types of tours available.

1. *Foreign clothing-optional beaches.* You can travel to a clothing-required resort that has a legal clothing-optional beach nearby. These resorts are located in places such as Europe, the Caribbean, and Tahiti. At most of these resorts (such as the Club Mediterranee in the Caribbean or Tahiti) clothing is required all the time except at the clothing-optional beach.

2. *Foreign nude resorts.* The concept of social nudism began in Europe, and nude resorts and beaches have been much more widely accepted there than in the United States; in fact, there are some six hundred camps and resorts in Europe. Germany has the most, and France is a close second. A popular nudist mecca is the Ile du Levant on the French Riviera, where both locals and visitors go around totally bare, except when within the confines of the village itself (on the dock, the streets and paths), where they wear *le minimum* (a small triangle of cloth covering the genitals and tied at the back with string). Yugoslavia has been wooing the tourist dollar by featuring nude resorts at reasonable rates.

3. *Nude cruises.* These cruises vary from 110-foot schooners (where the only time clothing is required is in port) to luxury liners (where clothing is worn for dining and dancing).

Like any other form of travel, nude travel provides fun, excitement, and the adventure of visiting foreign countries. It is travel with a plus, providing an opportunity to experience social nudity in new environments where the old social constraints seem far away and less compelling. Activities can take on new dimensions when done in the nude—scuba diving in the clear water of the Caribbean, for example. And the fact that a person is likely to be with strangers he will never see again makes nude travel an excellent way for first-timers to experience group nudity.

In the countries you visit, social nudity is not only accepted, but legal (in the United States, as mentioned, the legal status of nude beaches is still clouded). You have the maximum opportunity to make choices: whether you want to go nude or not, what you want to wear and when.

If you are totally unfamiliar with nudity, it is best to take a clothing-optional trip, rather than go to a nudist resort such as the Ile du Levant, where clothing would make you conspicuous. In fact, on a clothing-optional trip, you need never take your clothes off—nudity is permitted only at the nude beach, which you don't have to visit.

Some people are concerned that nude travel is a cover for orgies and mate-swapping. It is not. As with any travel, what people do in private cannot be regulated, but the social nudity you experience on a tour will be no less safe than going to a nude beach or resort in the United States.

Most tours do not have official leaders. Individuals purchase a packaged tour and go on their own. Some of the larger groups or some specialized tours have a manager who goes along, but his function is to handle the travel arrangements, not to make the trip a "meaningful" one in terms of social nudity. To date, Emily has conducted the only clothing-optional tour (to Tahiti in 1973) that had structured educational experiences included in the tour package. On this trip the participants had a chance to experiment with social nudity, if they desired, and also to learn about and try new methods for improving male-female relationships.

We believe the next trend in nude and clothed travel will be the addition of organized and structured types of learning experiences. They will be "living laboratories" for people who want to try new things in a new environment away from the pressures of job, home, and the people left behind.

There are a number of nudist travel clubs made up of people who meet regularly at nude resorts, beaches, or private homes. These people enjoy social nudity on a more organized basis than those who occasionally go to nude beaches or take nude trips. The advantage of belonging to a nude travel club is that it provides familiarity (members know each other), flexibility (members can participate in many activities from private parties to volleyball), and freedom (they are not restricted by so many rules as beach or camp nudists since they often meet in private homes).

For those interested in body liberation, it's worth taking a trip to a new kind of environment—to a growth center such as Esalen, Elysium, and Sandstone. Spending some time at these places will allow you to see yourself against a background as different from your own as a foreign culture. You can examine the values you have chosen to live by and learn about other values and behaviors that are open to you.

Chapter 13
Growth Centers: Esalen, Elysium, and Sandstone

> I'm glad that places such as Elysium and Sandstone exist and I'm sympathetic to their struggle, legal and otherwise, to survive. They serve a much needed purpose—for people to do some experimenting, stretching and exploring. I like it when the attitude of the growth center is "Hey, we are not happy with the system and our lives and so we are working out some new systems organizationally. If you'd like to try exploring with us, we'd like to have you." It is only when growth centers get righteous and say "we have found the way" that I object to them.
>
> Dr. Thomas Greening, editor of the
> *Journal of Humanistic Psychology*

Growth centers are educational institutions, but the education offered probably is unlike any you've ever had before. Growth centers focus on you as a total person—mind, body, and soul. You have an opportunity to incorporate into your lifestyle new information and ideas in a wide variety of fields (education, religion, medicine, sex, philosophy) and to experience and learn through your body as well as your mind. These centers offer a variety of courses and workshops in body knowledge areas—body image, sexuality, massage, holistic health, etc. Some incorporate nudity into their programs, providing various kinds of nude workshops or permitting participatory nudity in outdoor settings.

It is up to each participant to explore and take advantage of the resources of a growth center in his own way. There is no set curriculum; no formal structure dictates when he is ready to "graduate." Their innovative courses do not draw arbitrary distinctions between knowledge and experience or mind and body. They offer recreational facilities, places to stay overnight, beautiful gardens or other quiet places to meditate, and the chance to learn from highly respected professionals and innovators in many disciplines. Most important, today's new educational institutions offer an opportunity for participants to *grow*—to liberate themselves from rigid patterns of acting, thinking, and feeling.

There are many growth centers throughout the nation, but in this chapter we will describe three—Esalen (in Big Sur in Northern California) and Elysium Field and Sandstone Ranch (both in the Los Angeles area). Each is a prototype of a new concept in education. While each recognizes the importance of the mind-body unity, each center places its emphasis on a different aspect of this mind-body integration. At Esalen, for example, the focus is on discovering harmonious, humanistic, and healthful ways for people to learn, play, relate, love, and work by paying as much attention to their emotions and body sensations as to their thinking ability. At Elysium, the emphasis is on realizing body joy by shedding inhibiting and joy diminishing body taboos. A wide variety of body workshops and a beautiful, sensual atmosphere where the wearing of clothes is always optional helps the participants do just that. At Sandstone, the emphasis is on providing a "serene setting where the real worth and dignity of human sexuality may be experienced." Through structured and professionally led body-centered workshops and an atmosphere where open expressions of sexuality between consenting adults is permitted, participants are free to explore their own sexuality in ways that are growth-promoting and comfortable.

ESALEN

Esalen was founded in 1962 by Michael Murphy and Richard Price, Stanford University graduates who majored in philosophy and psychology. The simple, weather-stained one-story buildings that make up the center are located about one hundred miles south of San Francisco on a cliff overlooking the ocean. About fifty-five people—staff members and families—live there year round. Accommodations are comfortable but not lavish. Guests make their own beds, and the dining room is self-service. Guests are also asked to help out in the kitchen if they sign up for one of the special residential programs.

Esalen is a community where people can try new ways of relating and living. Traditional Western thought and ancient Eastern philosophies are practiced and combined with new theories in education, the behavioral and physical sciences, religion and philosophy. Work done at Esalen has made a substantial theoretical and practical contribution to what is often called the "new education," which considers feeling as important as rational thought and human interaction as important as factual knowledge. The new educational philosophy suggests, among other things, the practicing of non-competitive games, which stress fun and cooperation instead of struggle and winning, and holistic medicine.

About one hundred people go to Esalen each week to take the workshops, to enjoy a new sort of environment, and to experience the famous Esalen baths, which draw from some natural hot springs. The baths, which are housed in a building with a magnificent view of the sea, are built so that fifteen people can sit comfortably. In the baths, workshop participants meet for informal discussions and socializing. Strangers share feelings, talk about ideas, and touch each other physically and emotionally. And it is in the bathhouse that the massage perfected and made famous at Esalen is given—a technique that involves gentle stroking of all parts of the body except the genitals.

Nude mixed bathing is now taken for granted at Esalen although originally men and women stayed in their own sections of the bathhouse. It gradually became apparent that it was more natural for men and women to bathe together— couples wanted to be together, workshop participants who had grown close did not want to be separated during this frequently meaningful experience. Now whenever nudity seems appropriate and natural at Esalen—whether in the baths or the pool or on the massage tables—it takes place.

Esalen was the first educational establishment to permit mixed nude bathing. However, the focus at Esalen is not on nudity; people do not go into the dining room, attend workshops, or wander around the grounds nude.

Concern and respect for the human body is an important aspect of an Esalen education. There are several programs devoted to special kinds of body treatments. For example, there is a five-week course aimed at helping people stay well. This program—"The Inner Road to Health: Approaches to Healing and Self-Healing"—includes meditation, yoga, tai chi, jogging, occasional fasting, bioenergetics, and acupuncture, as well as lectures on such subjects as anatomy and physiology.

There are many other body-centered workshops, varying in length from a weekend to several weeks, which integrate the body therapies with other techniques and psychotherapies.

The learning process at Esalen is not always without pain. Learning is often an unsettling process because you have to take a look at your cherished assumptions and ask yourself challenging questions—questions for which there are no easy or pat answers. Because Esalen is a center for experimental education, only those with an educational intent are encouraged to visit. A person with severe emotional problems might find the experience upsetting, and the Esalen catalog specifically warns people not to come seeking a "cure."

Yet there seems to be something almost therapeutic in the Esalen environment itself. After the workshops, you can wander around absorbing the sights, sounds, and smells. You will neither have crowds of people to contend with, nor will you be left to sit alone and be lonely. Individuals gather in groups and then separate to try activities they may never have thought of trying or always wanted to try and never could: a teacher may try doing tai chi, a banker may try playing a flute, a pharmacist and his wife whose relationship has lost its zest may wrestle playfully in the pool.

The major contribution of Esalen to body liberation is in its creation of a climate for people to explore all aspects of their humanness, mental and physical. Another growth center, Elysium, is carrying the idea of body liberation a step further.

ELYSIUM FIELD

Like Esalen, Elysium Field is a growth center with many of the same kinds of educational programs. It is also a *sensual* spa, a place where, weather permitting, most people go nude most of the time.

Probably it is the attention paid to whatever delights the senses that most distinguishes Elysium both from other growth centers and from nude resorts. Located on an eight-acre site in Topanga Canyon (in Los Angeles), Elysium is at the end of an oak-lined country lane. The large wrought iron gate at the entrance is marked with a six-foot *ankh*, the ancient Egyptian talisman symbolizing eternal life and the merging of male and female. Also scattered around are outdoor metal sculptures of people dancing; brightly colored murals; wind chimes of shells, bronze, and glass. Inside the fence, a grassy hillside slopes down from an outdoor jacuzzi to a swimming pool surrounded by natural wood buildings. This green expanse forms the backdrop for a grape arbor, pebble paths, and flowering trees and shrubs, all carefully planted but casually arranged. No radios, television sets, or tape recorders are permitted at Elysium; you can hear goats, chickens, and horses from neighboring fields. There are no private rooms or cabins for overnight guests, but you can bring a sleeping bag or bedroll. You can sleep on the floor, dormitory style, in one of the large seminar rooms or outside on the grass.

On the grassy hillside people may be talking, napping, playing backgammon, massaging one another, strumming guitars. Children of all ages are welcome. People are usually nude, perhaps adorned with brightly colored scarves, hats, or jewelry. The people who go to Elysium are largely professionals—psychologists, teachers, doctors, executives, and so on.

Some men and women will be seen wearing loose, flowing India print robes when it gets chilly. Since discarding one's clothing is an option and not a rule, it is a violation of social custom to pressure those who have clothes on to disrobe. Usually, if Elysium members sense that people are newcomers—wearing clothes or not—they will try to strike up a conversation and make them feel comfortable.

At Elysium, people reach out to one another, and they openly take pleasure in looking at one another's bodies. The attitude is that bodies and their functions are wholesome. Indeed, it is the idea that *all parts* are wholesome, even sexual ones, that makes Elysium philosophically different from nudist camps. Sex education classes for adults, for example, are held in the nude and though no sexual intercourse is allowed, people talk about such taboo subjects as masturbation, sexual fantasies and fears, and anatomy. The aim is to expand one's repertoire of sexual behavior.

Elysium also differs from nudist camps in that most people who go there are interested in nudity not merely for the sake of nudity, but as a means of personal expression, as an option in behavior, and as a means of helping to develop a more natural lifestyle. Many are concerned with nutrition, and include in their diets fresh vegetables, organic foods, and whole-grain cereals, rather than calorie-laden desserts, potato chips, and soft drinks. Many are teetotalers or drink only small amounts of wine.

Body liberation at Elysium includes a deep concern that people do not get so bored and anxious during their leisure time that they hurt their bodies with drugs, alcohol, and improper diet. There are a number of programs designed to improve the quality of leisure time—to make it more emotionally nourishing and physically pleasurable.

Most at Elysium are much more comfortable with touching and being touched than the usual nudist. Touching is encouraged in many of the workshops and by the permissive Elysium atmosphere. However, since people are also encouraged to set their own limits, it is considered acceptable to discourage unwanted touching. Touching for the purpose of sexual arousal is expressly forbidden in public because of the presence of children. Friends may rub one another's bodies, including breasts and genitals, with suntan lotion or massage oil, but they are not permitted to fondle them in a sexually provocative way. However, there are two rooms—the "meditation rooms"—which have been set aside for people who want to be alone or who want privacy to make love.

Elysium differs from most other growth centers in its attitude toward bodily pleasure. It isn't that the other growth centers aren't interested in pleasure—they are, but their programs are frequently so solemn in nature that the search for joy can become a pretty ponderous business. Elysium presents programs that combine fun with education. Participants are taught to be childlike without being childish (that is, without being irresponsible, without violating the rights of others), and so they may romp in a huge mud puddle, feed one another, wash one another in the shower, or paint each other's bodies.

Elysium has a unique outlook on male-female relationships. Acknowledging the fact that single people are interested in meeting other single people, it has programs structured to help people find what they want, whether it is a date, a bed partner, or a lifetime mate. With the help of a skilled leader, ways of relating that are seldom seriously considered elsewhere are openly discussed here—things such as *ménage à trois*, multiple relationships, group marriage, bisexuality, and older women with younger men.

An Elysium Case History

Going to Elysium Field changed actor Dom DeLuise's attitude toward his own body. DeLuise went to Elysium for the first time on business—to interview "nudists in their own habitat" for a Steve Allen television show. Although DeLuise was initially reluctant, Allen convinced him he was the ideal person to do the show; as a "likeable performer" he would, while dressed, be able to candidly interview men, women, and children who were *not* dressed. After a lot of talking and negotiating, DeLuise agreed to do the show—but only if he could decide which film was going to be used or even if *any* was to be used.

Although DeLuise as a performer appreciated the challenge, privately he thought he was going into an "insane situation"—one where he would be interviewing people he didn't know, who were naked, while the camera was recording his every reaction for posterity. But once inside the gates of Elysium, he noticed something strange:

> The naked people were warm, communicative, relaxed, affectionate, and *calm*. In fact, the only calm people were the naked ones. The people wearing clothes—the cameraman, the director, the technicians—were so "up-

tight" they wanted me to have a drink with them for "strength." I refused on the grounds that if the people at Elysium could go naked without the aid of a drink, I could interview them without one."

The first person Dom met at Elysium was Emily, standing in the midst of a group of naked people, clothed more than most in a hat and two bracelets. Emily gave him a warm smile and a big hug as he was, he says, "trying desperately to look at the eyes of these naked people and appear cool." But as DeLuise interviewed the "naked people" and found them to be "just people" who happened to enjoy swimming, sunning, relaxing, reading, or even (in the case of one woman) vacuuming the living room in the nude, his fears turned to interest. He learned that many of these people had once been uptight about revealing their naked bodies to others for fear they would be rejected for some bodily imperfection. As a chronically overweight person, Dom had always been self-conscious about his body and even in his own home alone had felt gross and uncomfortable walking around naked.

Watching Emily conduct some tenderness-training and affection-sharing exercises with a group of men and women of all ages, DeLuise found that nudity and sexuality are not one and the same. Watching the participants sitting in a circle and touching the people near them—their arms, backs, faces—with gentle *awareness*, DeLuise said to Emily, "This is wonderful."

Emily looked into his eyes, slowly patted him on the shoulder and replied, "Thank you for being so human. When they said a comedian was going to come here to interview us, I was scared he was going to joke about us."

Dom was so touched that he cried. Then he called his wife, Carol, and told her he was experiencing something very special—something that was going to change his thinking in important ways.

Several weeks later DeLuise returned to Elysium alone and this time he shed his clothes. Afterwards he felt lighter and more comfortable with himself, despite his still overweight body: "The feeling of acceptance I got was wonderful. No one put any conditions on the acceptance of me—like we'll like you as soon as you lose ten pounds or anything. They saw me and thought of me as okay even if I am fat."

DeLuise wanted to share this wonderful new growth experience with Carol—even though the thought of her being able to compare his naked and overweight body to more conventionally pleasing male bodies made him feel threatened. Although Carol saw no sense in going to Elysium and although she was determined not to take off her clothes, because she loves him she agreed to go and to take their two young sons.

When they arrived, Dom took off his clothes and got into the jacuzzi while Carol and the children stayed dressed and watched. Soon it seemed silly to leave the children's clothes on, and so Carol undressed them and let them run around freely. Then it seemed even sillier to her to be the only one there with clothes on, so Carol undressed.

Dom experienced Carol's going with him to Elysium when she didn't want to, undressing when she didn't plan to, and still loving him in spite of the fact that she saw many trimmer male bodies as a tremendous act of love and acceptance. It helped bridge some minor tensions that had been interfering with their sex life, and that night there was a new passion between them which, in fact, resulted in the conception of their third son. In addition, the family learned to be easy about their nudity, whether bathing together or just sitting around the house.

SANDSTONE RANCH

At Elysium, nudity is permitted anywhere, anytime, but overt sexual behavior is limited. At Sandstone Ranch, on the other hand, not only is nudity permitted anywhere, anytime, but erotic sex play and sexual intercourse are permitted anywhere, anytime, so long as there has been mutual consent.

While sexual intercourse in front of others or group sex is obviously not the norm in American society, Sandstone was not founded on the whim of some sexual deviates. Inspired by a carefully planned vision of social reform, Sandstone's founders, Paul Paige, a psychotherapist, and Joel Scheinbaum, a psychiatrist, have private practices in Santa Monica, California. Paige believes that a center dedicated to sexual exploration must include structured and professionally led workshops, aesthetically beautiful and spotlessly clean surroundings, and perhaps most important of all, highly committed and responsible members.

Newcomers are impressed by the relaxed and serene atmosphere. The main structure, a low U-shaped ranch house, is built around an exquisite reflection pool, designed so that the slightest movement of the water causes the ringing of soft chimes.

Inside, the shag-carpeted living room is ringed with plush burnt-orange sofas which face the fireplace and a whole wall of glass. Outside the living room, there is a sundeck which overlooks a large expanse of lawn, and beyond that, in the distance, the ocean.

There are many things to do at Sandstone—dance, swim in the Olympic-sized swimming pool, soak in the jacuzzi, play ping-pong, enjoy a gourmet dinner, watch feature-length films relevant to the human potential movement. Although most people are nude, there are usually some people dressed in long robes or street clothes.

It is not easy to gain admittance to Sandstone. At this writing there are three types of participation—the "intentional family" of approximately fourteen people who live and work cooperatively at Sandstone, the members who go to Sandstone to take advantage of the usual and unusual recreational activities, and workshop participants who go there for the educational benefits. Members and guests who attend the social events must be accompanied by a partner of the opposite sex because of the center's desire to keep a balance of the sexes.

How are the activities at Sandstone "educational"? Although sex is one of the most important human activities, most people never see others engaged in sexual intercourse except in pornographic movies—and these usually give a distorted view of sexual organs and sexual acts, never showing the tender, human side of sexual activities. Most people never get a chance to learn from others or to try out their sexual fantasies in a supportive atmosphere. The center rejects the philosophy that the main purpose of sex is procreation, that sex without love is harmful, that couples will automatically learn how to pleasure each other sexually. The center supports the idea that it is acceptable to have sex with a person one finds attractive but does not necessarily love. Sex for the sake of giving and getting pleasure presents some interesting learning possibilities. In order to have pleasurable sex with different temporary partners, a person must learn to communicate—to tell them what he or she wants and to find out what they want. (Learning to communicate can also improve sex with one's permanent partner.)

People who feel restricted by sexual convention might be interested in learning about Sandstone's philosophy and how it affects the lives of individuals. Sandstone offers workshops with such titles as "The Lovemaking Experience," "Enriching Sexuality Through Hypnosis," "Expression Through Movement and Intimacy." Sandstone also has an experimental research program called "The Enhancement of Sexual Functioning," which is based on the assumption that everyone can learn more, regardless of present skills, abilities, and levels of functioning—both as an individual and as a partner in an intimate relationship.

You need not attend a structured program to have an educational and liberating experience at Sandstone. For example, you can attend a social evening, with or without participating in sexual activity. In fact, sometimes a major educational benefit is the realization that you don't *have to* participate sexually—you can observe and learn and satisfy your curiosity without being pressured into doing something you don't want to do.

Sandstone, on any Wednesday or Saturday night, at first glance appears to be an ordinary social situation, except for the nudity. Men and women are talking, laughing, flirting, or sitting quietly together. Like Elysium, there is a lot of affectionate touching; unlike Elysium, you might see a man and woman sitting in front of the fireplace fondling each other's genitals. Erotic play is allowed everywhere, but most of the sexual activity at Sandstone takes place in what is jokingly called the "ball room," a small room with wall-to-wall mattresses covered with clean fitted sheets.

At Sandstone, people are as free to ask others to have sex with them as they would be to ask them to dance. There is also complete freedom to decline. It is taken for granted that women enjoy sex, and that they can and should ask for it when they want it, without fear of being thought less feminine. It is also taken for granted that men *don't* want sex sometimes. What is surprising to most people is the quiet and easy flowing of the sexual encounters at Sandstone. One sees much tenderness and playfulness. The pushing, grabbing, anxious, impulsive, orgiastic sex pictured in pornographic movies is absent.

Many people have a feeling that good sex is in short supply. They worry about two things: "Am I ever going to get enough sex?" "Am I going to have an orgasm?" At Sandstone, a person can fulfill (or try to fulfill) his fantasy of unlimited sex and, in time, in such a sexually permissive atmosphere, he will find he can be more selective and more relaxed.

Without inner awareness, a sexually permissive atmosphere can be the loneliest place in the world—a place where bodies touch in a meaningless way. Those who have sex without awareness, divorce the body from the mind. The high degree of self-awareness possessed by many Sandstone members keeps it from being a swingers club. While sex without commitment is the norm at Sandstone, sex without interpersonal involvement is not the norm. Most people are seeking better relationships; they want to touch another person—emotionally, sexually, intellectually—if only for a while.

An interesting aspect of Sandstone is what it can do for the many married or otherwise committed couples who go there. Sandstone assumes that it is a fact of human nature that people like variety—that, like a straight diet of steak and mushrooms, even good sex with someone you love can become a bore after a while. Eventually boredom saps the life from a relationship or else one or both partners secretly play around and *guilt* saps the life from the relationship. At Sandstone it is possible to have variety by having sex with others openly, without making rash promises or feeling guilty. Or one can add variety to his or her sexual life by taking classes, observing others, and learning new techniques and methods of communication.

THE FUTURE OF GROWTH CENTERS

Growth centers are increasing, not only in numbers, but in variety. Although there are more in California than in any other state, they can be found in almost every part of the United States—and in other countries as well. (See our list of addresses at the end of the book for information on how to locate a growth center near you.) Growth centers have already had a significant impact on the lives of many people and will become even more influential in the future. Just as it has long been commonplace for people to attend week-long out-of-town conferences, weekend workshops, or weekly night classes to enhance their vocational skills and keep up with what is going on in their professions, it will soon become equally commonplace for people to go to growth centers for a day, a weekend, or several weeks to bring their energies and their lives into balance. Just as people have always sought specialized kinds of educational institutions to meet their needs (adult education centers, college extension divisions, universities, law schools, real estate schools, and so forth) they are now seeking specialized kinds of growth centers.

In addition to the kinds of centers we have discussed in this chapter, there are centers that focus on meditation, on helping people make life changes they want to make or have to make (such as retirement, divorce, death of a loved one), on teaching nutrition and exercise.

There is a need for another kind of growth center, one where people can go just to play with other people at a time when they are seeking fun more than learning—a place to be rejuvenated, revitalized, refreshed. People need a place that will provide and encourage new kinds of play and socialization—a kind of play-oriented growth center that could properly be called a holistic vacation resort.

New kinds of places to play are needed because as people become more and more integrated, mind and body, the kind of escapist activities that are hard on the mind, the body, and the pocketbook interest them less and less. A vacation of dissipation—overeating, drinking, gambling, running from one place to another, or overexercising—is not what they seek. Emily hopes someday to develop such a center, a center where she can provide the same sort of holistic vacation experience she provided for the participants on her two-week "Learning While Playing" holiday in Tahiti in 1973.

The learning part of the holiday centered around Emily's workshop on "Making Friends with the Opposite Sex." The "playing" centered around the activities at the Club Mediterranee in Tahiti. However, as with all of Emily's workshops, it soon became impossible to distinguish between the learning and the playing. Four times a week an outrigger canoe took Emily and the participants to a private island where the workshop was held. The privacy and the beautiful weather resulted in the participants spontaneously asking if they could be nude during the workshop. After verifying that no participant objected, Emily agreed and the workshop became clothing-optional.

The workshop participants, though outnumbered ten to one by the other guests at Club Med, soon improved the mood of the entire group. Even one or two of them at a dinner table, in the cocktail lounge, in an outrigger, or in the water-skiing and snorkeling classes made a difference in the ease with which the others talked and treated each other. The workshop participants' joyousness and comfort with themselves and others spread in all directions.

Just as this new type of vacation experience is developing because of the need for health-promoting, body-appreciating forms of fun and relaxation, so new forms of at-home socializing are beginning to develop. After all, it isn't sensible to limit your body joy and fun to two weeks a year or to the times you can go to a nude beach or growth center. One of the major benefits of body liberation, in fact, is the discovery that enjoying your body can be an ongoing process, one you can share with friends in your own home. The next chapter is about a new sort of party that promotes body joy and closer relationships with your friends.

Chapter 14
Body Joy with Others

> I believe that in the future not only will special nudist communities like Elysium increase, but that social nudism at home—between parents and children and close friends of the family—will be more common. I think this is almost inevitably going to happen because of the growing feelings of candor, directness, honesty, freedom, and a new willingness to affirm that the human body is a very beautiful thing.
>
> Max Lerner,
> columnist for the *New York Post*

This chapter is primarily about body parties—new ways of socializing that focus on fun, relaxation, and interpersonal closeness through activities that promote body joy. We will describe in detail a unique kind of body-joy party that we gave, one that permitted, even encouraged, nudity.

Perhaps you are now saying, "Okay, Emily and Betty, this time you've gone too far. Most of the suggestions up to now have been ones I could see some sense in, even if I didn't want to try them. But if being liberated or having fun means I have to give a nude party for my friends, forget it." Let us reassure you that our body party is *not* being presented as a necessary step to body liberation. Liberating your body is a continuing process that is individual to you and does not depend on how many activities you participate in or in what order. Our purpose is to suggest some new ways of behaving with your friends in your own home that can enhance your friendships and make body joy available to you on a year-round, inexpensive basis. We hope that many of you, after reading this chapter and laughing a little at our party, will be stimulated enough to dream up some ideas of your own to promote body-joy experiences with your friends. Sharing pleasure is one of the best ways of getting close to others, and body joy is a basic form of pleasure, one that can cement long-standing friendships and quickly start new ones.

We suspect, that while many of you may want to have a body party (some we'll describe don't require disrobing and are so proper that your Aunt Mabel could attend), not many will want to give a party like ours. But just as you enjoy watching a travelogue about a place you never intend to visit, chances are you'll enjoy reading about our unconventional nude social event.

Before we tell you about what we did at our party, we want to tell you what motivated us to give our first body party. We had body therapy, psychotherapy, been Rolfed, Feldenkraised, and Alexandered, spent time at growth centers, visited nude beaches, camps, and resorts. Though we had learned a lot, met wonderful people, and enjoyed ourselves along the way, to get our lives in better balance, we needed to play.

Though we get invited to many parties, few of them are much fun. It isn't because of a lack of food or drink—at most parties people eat and drink too much. Good people are at the parties we go to but they are frequently overconcerned with how they look or whether they are acting in an acceptable manner. Men and women are seldom able to be really comfortable with each other and their tension is evident in a nervous kind of flirting, dirty jokes, and *double entendres.* People stand around and talk and joke as if waiting for the party to begin, and we get the feeling that if we laugh too loud or dare to do anything different, we'll be out of place. After many such parties, we concluded that not only didn't we have much fun, but we didn't really make any meaningful contact with anyone.

OUR BODY-JOY PARTY

We decided that a body-joy party, one that encouraged people to appreciate their bodies and revel in their senses, was just what we needed. We believed we could design one that would avoid the usual social pitfalls, one that would give people an opportunity to shed their social tensions and inhibitions, to reveal themselves as they really are to each other—one that would encourage laughter, affection, and creativity.

We thought the option of nudity would add to the fun. However, we also knew that the option to disrobe would not, of itself, help people relax and interact; we have been to nude parties that were not much fun—for all the same reasons that make most clothed parties boring. To make our party different we knew we had to create a friendly, non-critical atmosphere and help people interact in ways that would relieve their stress about status and roles. We wanted an atmosphere that would encourage people to express themselves spontaneously—to speak up, move, laugh, and touch.

This was quite an assignment we gave ourselves, but the challenge intrigued us. Within a week, our plans were laid and the following invitations were in the mail.

EMILY AND BETTY
are having a
CLOTHING-OPTIONAL PARTY

Date: February 7, 1976

Time: Please arrive between 6:30 and 7:00 PM. We are going to start introductions and activities at 7:00 PM—*on the dot.*

Bring: Sensual food for a "Tom Jones" dinner—something that looks, smells, and tastes good and can be served and eaten with the fingers.

Scarves, jewelry, and if possible, pieces of cloth large enough to wrap around you.

What to
Expect: Some interesting people, some unusual activities. (However, there will be no sex and no alcohol—just fun.)

The phone began ringing a few days after our invitation went out. Our invitees wanted to know more.

Would they be expected to go nude? No.

How come there would be no alcohol? We want people to be able to cope with their nervousness without artificial help, we said, so that their heads will be clear and they will know what they are doing.

Could they bring a friend or a date? No. For this experimental evening we only want people we know well.

As we discussed our party with our potential guests, we tried to dispel their fears about a clothing-optional party. We made it clear that nothing embarrassing was going to happen. We knew that most of our friends weren't likely to come unless we assured them that the nudity would not lead to sex. We let them know there would be fun, knowledge, a chance to meet new and interesting people.

The Guest List

We spent more time on our guest list than on anything else. A body-joy party presents an excellent opportunity to break with conventional social structuring, including a "couples only, same age" kind of set-up. We had an opportunity to invite people as individuals, not worrying about the male-female guest ratio or age similarities—variety makes a party more interesting. We wanted people who were not necessarily familiar with nudity, but who were intrigued at exploring new ideas.

Not everyone accepted. In fact, we got turned down by some of the very people we thought would be most enthusiastic. One bachelor said he could imagine a party without the possibility of sex but not one without liquor. A liberal lawyer didn't think his wife could handle it. A beautiful young woman thought being nude or partially undressed in the presence of men she didn't know would invite unwelcome sexual advances and yet felt she could not keep her clothes on if others disrobed. Another woman who had had a mastectomy was also apprehensive about the idea of social nudity, even if it was optional.

Though we had not intended a couples party, we had planned on a roughly even balance of men and women. However, we wound up with nine men and six women (including ourselves). The male guests included a minister, dentist, certified public accountant, men's clothing salesman, foundry owner, industrial psychologist, personnel manager, realtor, and geologist. The occupations of the women were elementary school principal, vocational counselor, housewife, and secretary. We had one married couple—the minister and his wife.

Since our party was meant to be a group as well as an individual experience, we told everyone to be on time. We knew that if people followed their ordinary party behavior (arriving whenever convenient or being "fashionably" late) we might not be able to build the group rapport necessary for this kind of party.

The Planning

We carefully planned for contact-making and comfort-building activities that would involve the guests as soon as they arrived. We knew the kind of emotional mood we wanted to create and got to work creating it. Most hosts and hostesses spend many hours planning for a party—determining the food and table settings, getting the house and yard in shape, and so on. Few plan activities that will help their guests get to know each other better. To some, the idea of planning any activity at all seems too calculated; they would rather rely on social spontaneity—which may or may not happen.

We felt we had to help our guests get started on the activities at our body party. To make it easy, we first took all of the furniture out of the living room and replaced it with an oval of brightly colored mats and sofa pillows. We wanted people to be able to lounge on the floor, yet be able to see everyone else.

In two of the bedrooms, we put out supplies for a dress-up game. For our Tom Jones dinner, instead of using a table we put a plastic dropcloth covered with a paper tablecloth on the rug in the family room. Because there is nothing worse than cool rooms or cold furniture at a nude party, we heated the rooms well in advance and had plenty of wood available for the fireplace.

Shortly before the guests arrived we dimmed all the lights (but not too dim, since we did not want to suggest an erotic atmosphere). We also lit candles in every room and saw to it that soft music was playing.

One person who had declined our invitation accused us of overplanning: "If nudity is so natural, how come you natural nudists need so many rules?" Our structure and rules were designed not to keep people in line, but to allow them to feel safe and comfortable enough to try something as unfamiliar as social nudity. We knew that some careful structuring was needed if we were to create *more* joy and spontaneity than is apparent at most traditional parties.

The Arrival

As the guests arrived and after the usual kissing and handshaking, we gave each person a cup of spiced cider, since we knew most persons feel uncomfortable at the beginning of a party and don't quite know what to do with their hands. We also gave them name tags in spite of objections like, "Hey what do we do with the tag when we take off our clothes?"

There were two reasons for the name tags. We knew they would reduce anxiety since many people don't talk with or look at people they don't know. And perhaps more important was the easy touching of hostess and guest as the name tag was applied. Many guests are afraid of body contact, but contact by a host or hostess at the beginning of a party helps them feel grounded, makes them feel arrived and safe. After a while each guest was asked to take off his or her shoes and sit on the pillows on the floor in such a way that he could see every other guest. Then Emily welcomed our guests: "Betty and I want to welcome you and thank you for agreeing to come to such an unusual sort of party. We think you'll find it not only worthwhile but a lot of fun. All of you were invited because you are interesting, open-minded people we enjoy being with. We think you'll enjoy being with each other even though many of you are still just getting acquainted."

Emily then talked about some of the fears people have about going nude for the first time with other people (we discussed these in Chapter 10). She asked if anyone would like to tell what he was feeling at the moment. After some lighthearted comments from our guests, many of whom admitted to having some apprehensions, we proceeded to our first activity.

The Conceal-Reveal Game

We asked our guests to think about the clothing they had chosen to wear to the party, saying clothing reveals a lot about our attitudes toward our bodies. We use clothing, for example, to show off bodily features we particularly like. The woman who always wears short skirts probably likes her legs and the man who wears tight tank-tops most likely admires the bulging biceps he is revealing. Clothing emphasizes our sexuality. (As discussed previously clothing may be more erotic than nudity.)

We also use clothing to conceal—both what we see as outer physical defects *and* our inner feelings. We camouflage ourselves with make-up and clothes—sometimes adding dark glasses, beards, and bulky outer garments so that no one can really tell who we are and what we are feeling. Probably our discomfort with nudity stems not only from the exposure of our genitals but also from the exposure of feelings we prefer to keep hidden.

We sometimes seem to take on the characteristics of the clothes we wear. For example, a softly-draped gown gives the body flexibility and grace; a steel helmet, leather jacket, gloves, and boots encase the wearer in a secure "cocoon"; and a long-trailing robe forces a person to move his body with regal dignity. Certainly the clothing of the Victorians contributed to their reputation as "strait-laced" and "stiff-necked." How could they possibly have been playful or sensuous in clothing that kept their bodies in upright and unyielding postures?

Explaining that it can be fun to discover what our clothing choices say about our attitudes and that it can also help us get to know each other better, Emily gave directions for a game called "Conceal-Reveal." Each participant has a chance to talk, uninterrupted, about what he or she has chosen to wear and why. Touching something he is wearing, the participant is to say whether he wears it because it covers up some part of his body he is not proud of, or because it shows off something he is proud of. He then takes off an item of clothing or jewelry, puts it in the center of the circle, and tells the group what facet of him it represents and how he feels after removing it.

Dressed in a silky, slinky, sleeveless copper-colored pants suit accented with jangling gold earrings, chains, and bracelets, Emily starts the game by following her own instructions: "I'm wearing this blouse because it covers up my fat stomach. I'm also wearing it because it shows off my breasts and small waist. This blouse, which is silky and smooth, represents my sensuous side—I like to run my hands down my body and feel the silkiness. It fits close to my body across my chest but flares out over my hips and stomach." She then removed the top. "I feel good now," she went on. "I like my body and I like the way these gold chains look on my bare breasts. I like to wear jewelry when I don't have clothes on."

When she finished, Emily flipped a coin to see whether the person on her left or right would go next. The accountant, a bachelor who was wearing a royal blue knitted sport shirt and closely fitted corduroy trousers said, "I'm wearing these trousers because they cover up my genitals and legs. I really hate wearing trousers. I only wear them because it is a social convention, and I'd get arrested if I didn't. In my office I've even taken off my trousers while working. If my secretary ever came in unexpectedly I'd be in trouble. I guess I'm wearing this shirt because it shows off my chest. It is fitted and I like the way my arms look in the short sleeves. I don't wear longsleeved shirts and ties—that really makes me feel stuck in the image of the white-collar worker. With my sport shirt I can somehow maintain the illusion that I am my own man—a natural man. I guess the shirt represents the real me." He took off his trousers, revealing a pair of bright red shorts. "I really feel great now, like at home," he said. "Now I know for sure I'm not working."

The vocational counselor looked smashing in an embroidered Guatemalan dress and exotic Indian jewelry. "I'm wearing this loose dress with long stockings underneath. It covers up my entire body. I'm not feeling well tonight, and I need to be warm and protected. I feel like I'm all curled up inside my clothes like a cat. I'm wearing these earrings because they show off my face. I feel absolutely naked without earrings and I never go anywhere without them. They dangle against my ears and make me look dramatic." She took off one earring. "I feel awful now," she said, "like a part of me is missing."

After everyone had a turn we were an unusual looking group—Emily was topless except for her gold chains; the C.P.A. was trouserless; everyone else was missing something they had come with—tie, coat, shoes and socks, jewelry, or belt—all of which were piled in the middle of the room.

Emily next asked what we had thought about while doing the exercise, what we had noticed and felt. There was a ten-minute discussion, during which we realized that our comments on clothing revealed a lot about individual values. Emily then interrupted to say that although there were probably enough new things to think about and talk about to keep us going all evening, there was something else to do before supper. "We want to give you," she said, "the option to take off as much more of what you are wearing as you want to, and we've invented another little game to make it easy and fun."

The Undressing Option

Since our party was an evening indoor social event, and not the kind of situation where going bare might seem natural (such as a daytime swimming party), we had given a lot of attention to this stage of our party. Nudity that is not accompanied by rational choice and the feeling that one is doing what is appropriate and right is not liberating—indeed, it can lead to a lot of guilt feelings.

We knew we had to come up with a technique that would help people who chose to shed their clothes do so in as unself-conscious a manner as possible. Our solution was an exercise we lightly called "To Strip or not to Strip." Its purpose was threefold: (1) to allow people to choose how much of themselves, both body and psyche, they wanted to expose; (2) to eliminate the need for separate dressing rooms, which smacked of sneaking off to do something one felt guilty about doing; and (3) to defuse any sexual connotations of watching each other undress.

Since we also wanted to test our theory that such party games could successfully be introduced by any adventurous host or hostess, not only by someone with Emily's specialized background, Betty led the activity: "This is a clothing-optional party, and we want to reassure you that we mean the word optional literally. You are free to take off all your clothes, some of your clothes, or none of your clothes. Do what you really feel like doing. Whatever you choose, we'll give you lots of support and hope you'll do the same for each other."

Everyone was then asked to stand in a circle facing each other, then to turn around so that they could not see anyone else and to take off (or not take off) whatever articles of clothing they wanted. They were asked not to joke or talk or peek, but to concentrate on doing exactly what they wanted to do and on what they thought would happen as a result.

During the next few minutes, we heard sighs, muted giggles, buckles opening, zippers coming unzipped, and articles of clothing dropping to the floor. When there was only expectant silence, Betty asked everyone to turn around and sit down. "To Strip or not to Strip" produced some surprises. The clothing salesman who had joked about being eager for the "unveiling" had taken off only his shirt and socks. The minister who had needed considerable reassurance just to get him to agree to come to the party stood in unabashed glory in leopard-skin patterned bikini briefs. The vocational counselor had taken off her other earring and her Guatemalan robe and was standing in only her bra, half-slip, and stockings. The secretary had taken off a little bolero but was still fully dressed in blouse and pants. Betty had taken off everything.

Before going around the room and asking each person why he or she took off or left on particular garments or jewelry, and how they felt at the moment, Betty said, "I took off everything, even my rings and jewelry, because I want to be accepted for my unadorned self. I didn't used to like my body, but now I'm realizing my body is me. I'd even like to scrub off the makeup I put on earlier; suddenly it seems phony and unreal. Right now I am feeling like myself—comfortable sitting here and letting you see me as I am—no pretenses or cover-ups. It feels good to be able to do that."

The clothing salesman said, "I took off my shirt and socks, but I just couldn't go any further. I've never been nude before in public and I got the awful feeling that if I took off all my clothes the rest of you would be fully clothed and staring at me like I was an idiot. I'm feeling relieved right now that some of you are partly dressed too."

The dentist announced: "Well, I thought I would make this whole undressing procedure easier by wearing only a long robe with nothing on underneath. So I didn't have much choice. As you can see, I took my robe off. I did not take off my watch—I'm going to keep it on and ignore it—I'm tired of being ruled by time. At work, I have to keep on schedule with my patients. Right now, I'm feeling good for two reasons. One, I allowed myself to wear a long robe; I've never worn one before and I understand it makes me look like a guru. At first I thought people would think I wasn't masculine or something, but then I decided my masculinity doesn't hinge on what I am wearing. The second reason I feel okay is that I like my body. It isn't perfect but it has been good to me for forty-two years, even if I haven't always been good to it."

The level of relaxation in the group went up appreciably at the end of this game. The decision to dress or undress, the moment of truth, was over, and it had been a lot less traumatic than many had expected. Everyone started talking excitedly to people who had been strangers an hour earlier, sometimes hugging or patting one another with genuine affection. We then all turned toward preparing the food everyone had brought for the Tom Jones dinner, bustling about Betty's small kitchen, bumping into one another's naked or semi-naked bodies while preparing bowls and trays of food.

The "Tom Jones" Dinner

Our Tom Jones dinner was designed to allow our guests to express the joyous feelings welling-up in them as they experienced the freedom of shedding their usual party personalities along with their clothes. Inspired by the uninhibited eating scene in the movie *Tom Jones*, in which Tom and a woman companion shared a meal in a very uninhibited and sensuous way, these unusual dinners provide an opportunity for people to dispense with traditional (and inhibiting) table manners and create a new sort of etiquette—one that encourages fun, interaction, and comfort.

We encouraged our guests to dispense with traditional table manners—to feed each other, not to use napkins (licking their own and even other people's fingers), and in other ways to use food to make contact with others. Moreover, we urged our guests to feed *all* the senses—to enjoy the sight, smell, taste, sound, and feel of food in many different forms. There were finger foods—chicken legs, celery, crackers, cheese, fruit, asparagus tips—as well as dishes for the more adventurous to scoop up in handfuls—a noodle casserole, cottage cheese, Jello.

Typically at a Tom Jones dinner, conversation is forbidden and all communication takes place without words, through eye, hand, and body gestures. However, we knew there would be rebellion if we tried to impose silence on our guests who were feeling very friendly towards and curious about each other. The conversations were spontaneous and open because people—though mostly strangers at the beginning of the evening—already felt more comfortable with each other than they felt with some of their old friends. They felt released to do what they wanted to do—to be playful, to try behavior foreign to their image. The accountant playfully tossed olives and purple grapes across the table to the vocational counselor, who tried to catch them in her mouth. She decided, after a few grapes landed on her underwear, to shed the last of her clothes, declaring that it would be easier to launder a grape-stained body. Some felt free to dramatize themselves. For example, the dentist walked around offering a half watermelon filled with fruit compote, bowing from the waist like a slave at a Roman feast. Some lost the customary decorum of their roles in the outside world—the minister scooped up food in his hands and playfully fed his wife; the school principal poured pineapple juice in her navel. Some adapted their customary roles to these circumstances: the secretary surrounded herself with cheese covered crackers and, like a mother bird feeding her young, popped crackers into the mouths of the other guests.

The Fashion Show

Our guests discovered that being freed from traditional social rules and regulations did not lead to behavior that made them uncomfortable but to a sense of being involved with others in an enjoyable way. We capitalized on this mood for our next game. After dinner was cleared away and everyone washed up, we announced it was time for the dress-up fashion show.

The purpose of this activity is to encourage guests to reclaim the pleasure of decorating and displaying their bodies as they did as children. We divided the guests into two groups, each including both men and women, with Betty captaining one and Emily the other, and explained that each team would give a fashion show for the other. The reason for having the teams is to develop camaraderie and a cooperative spirit within each group, and to give purpose for individuals to strut and preen and display themselves for the others.

Each group went into a bedroom where supplies had been laid out: scarves, stoles, pieces of cloth, jewelry, belts, ribbons, bows, feathers, safety pins, scotch tape, and so on. Guests were also free to try out each other's clothing. We captains then instructed our team members to dress up in the way they'd like to dress if there were no rules that implied one part of the body is bad and must be covered and that another is good and can be uncovered. In this game, we said, all parts of the body are good and it is okay to show off, to apply your fantasies and creativity.

We set a twenty-minute deadline for getting dressed. The time limit facilitated cooperation. Some people asked others for help in getting the right drape of material over a shoulder or across the hips. Some requested assistance in taping bows to their bodies. And everyone wanted advice on how to make their costumes more attractive and original.

Betty's group, which went first, had opted to do a traditional fashion show complete with commentator—the secretary, now wearing the dentist's long robe, some fancy earrings, and an old-fashioned bonnet she had created. As the models paraded, they were received with laughter and applause. The previously modest clothing salesman brought down the house with his harem costume, which consisted of several sheer chiffon scarves covering him from head to toe—except for his eyes—and a decorative bow on his penis. The accountant did a jungle dance around the room, showing off his beaded loincloth and feathered anklets. The vocational counselor wore a colorful piece of cloth which covered her pubic region but not her breasts or buttocks, elbow-length white gloves, bows on her toes, and a peacock feather in her hair.

Emily's group was equally innovative. The industrial psychologist appeared as Sir Lance-a-Little in a Cossack-style fur hat, beaded belt with a knife in it, and boots. The minister shed the last of his ministerial dignity when, wearing a feathered headdress and not much else, he dashed into the room uttering an Indian war whoop. Emily walked on as Scarlett O'Hara, sporting an elegant white hat with flowers on it, a gold chain over her waist and hips, long earrings, gloves, and high heels.

Our guests loved the chance to show-off their bodies. During the fashion show the laughter level rose about two decibels and the guests were on a natural, joyous "high." This would have been a good time for spontaneous conversation and dancing. However, since this was an experimental evening, we were anxious to test all our activities. Therefore, we asked our guests to participate in one last activity—a group massage.

The Von Newman Massage and the End of the Party

During this massage, developed by group leader Stan Russell, one person lies on his stomach on a mat or towel while several others distribute themselves around his body—for example, one at his head, one on each side of the upper back and one on each side of the lower body. The massage is a carefully structured one requiring a leader, who at our party was Emily. During it, there is to be no giggling, tickling, funny remarks or erotic play. The massage finally gave the last holdout, the secretary, a *reason* to take off all her clothes. She was not about to miss the pleasures of being stroked gently on her back by several sets of loving hands. Although it took a long time, we saw to it that every person had a chance to enjoy this loving experience. (It takes about 20-30 minutes for each person.)

Emily instructed everyone that simultaneous placement of hands on and off the body of the person being massaged was very important. Although their touch should be firm but not heavy, the moment of first contact and withdrawal should be so gentle as to be barely perceptible. As everyone watched her, Emily raised her hands in the air and then lowered them as the signal for the others to make contact with the body being massaged. Three guests sighed happily as their massage-mates made contact with their bodies for about thirty seconds until Emily gave the signal for them to remove their hands.

In a very soft but authoritative voice Emily then said:

We are now going to touch our friend with the palms of our hands, fingers held close together, with a gentle slapping motion. Do not slap to make noise but to stimulate all of his body surfaces. Be sure to neglect no parts of him. Remember the sides of his body, his head, arms, and the soles of his feet. Let us now begin.

After about twenty seconds, Emily instructed:

Now speed up the pace. Go all over his body quickly and lightly. Now go slower and slower and lighter and lighter and now gradually stop.

At the end of this technique Emily signaled for everyone to withdraw hands and await instructions for the next method of contact.

There are a variety of other contact techniques but the basic method is always the same. Massagers touch the subject's body with the palms of their hands for about thirty seconds. Then hands are simultaneously lifted until instructions are given for the next technique. The following are the remaining means of contact and their proper sequence.

1. *Raindrops.* Fingertips touch and leave the body in rapid succession, like a spring rain, for about fifteen to twenty seconds.

2. *Fists.* Body is gently—very gently—pounded with everyone's fists for about fifteen to twenty seconds.

3. *Lotion application.* Group members hold out their hands, palms up, and the leader pours out a large quantity of lotion in one palm of each. Group members then pour the lotion back and forth from one palm to another several times, thus warming it to body temperature. Then all group members at once apply lotion in generous amounts with long,

sweeping motions to cover all parts of the body, including toes, neck, fingers, sides of the body, etc.

4. *Blowing.* All members bend down and blow their warm breath all over the body to dry the lotion.

5. *"Ohm-ming."* With all hands on the subject, group members say "ohm" in loud, clear voices, holding each "ohm" in a hum at the end for as long as possible, letting vibrations go from their throats through their hands into the body of their friend. This is repeated three times in succession.

6. *Peacock feathering.* The leader gives a peacock feather to each group member, and altogether they brush the subject's entire body with the tips of the soft feathers for about fifteen to twenty seconds. (Fur can be substituted if feathers aren't available.)

7. *Kissing.* All group members bend over their friend and shower his entire body with kisses, being sure to include the kissing of his cheeks, his ears, his buttocks and the bottom of his feet.

After fifteen seconds or so of kissing, Emily signals to the group members to cease. She leans down and whispers into the subject's ear:

> What you are now experiencing is reality. Lie there and enjoy reality as long as you care to. Then sit up and join us, but do so at your own pace. Take your time. You have all the time in the world.

As the group members wait for the "massagee" to stir, all sit quietly together, letting the quality of the shared silence penetrate. After each guest rouses himself, taking all the time he needs, another person is selected for the next round of Von Newman contact techniques.

A group massage is an emotionally powerful experience—a laying-on-of-hands that is healing, nourishing, tender, playful, and sensuous. At the end of the evening all of us gathered in friendly clusters in the dimly lit living room, sitting together in silence, savoring the closeness. People smiled softly, hugged, and touched. Some had tears in their eyes. At 2:00 A.M. our guests slowly departed, obviously tired but exhilarated, reluctant to sever the strong bond that had developed. And we, happy with our party, didn't even mind the cleaning up.

OUR CRITIQUE

The evening showed us that it is not only possible to get nice, cold-sober people to attend a party they know will include nudity, but also to get them to participate in activities that may at first seem inane and childish. In fact, after the party we were besieged with phone calls from people who had either refused our invitation or had not been invited; they wanted to know when we were going to give another party and whether they could please come. We said we couldn't possibly do all the body-party giving but that we would write up our party so they could give one of their own and invite us. The comments and suggestions we got from our guests were invaluable in helping us evaluate our party and plan future ones.

Most of our guests felt the experience had not only been a joyful one but also a consciousness-raising one. Here are some of their comments:

> I thought the dress-up contest was lots of fun. We got to know each other and had lots of laughs while we were being creative. Sticking a scarf on bare skin with scotch tape is certainly different.

> The Von Newman massage was terrific. It gave a beautiful finishing touch to the evening.

> The structure added to the relaxing of tensions. And I think nudity gave extra excitement to an already stimulating party.

We feel the major contribution to the party's success was the body-liberating, body-joy-promoting structure, rather than the fact that clothing was optional. People felt free enough to have body contact, to express their emotions, to try out new ways of behaving, to drop their social roles and be themselves, and to experience bodily pleasure without guilt. In a single evening some guests cast off inhibitions of a lifetime—inhibitions they had thought were permanent.

We suspect one reason people can shed the inhibitions that put barriers between them and other people so easily at times is that they are hungry for real contact with other people. No matter how much a person socializes, how many friends he has, how many parties he attends, chances are he doesn't often have the opportunity to reveal himself to others as he really is and to be accepted. The joy we observed in others and felt in ourselves at the party was the joy of people who had gotten in touch with their bodies and each other—the joy of people who had broken through social barriers to discover that their options for friendship and bodily pleasure are endless.

Ironically, our very success in helping people relate in such a joyful and open manner brought us a little bit of criticism from our guests who felt that they didn't have enough time to do some of the things they felt free enough to try. For example, some had felt so exhilarated after the dress-up game that they wanted to dance or play with some of the "toys" we had provided (jacks, jump ropes, balls, paints, batacas, etc.). Others wanted to have quiet one-to-one conversations with the people they had grown close to in the course of the evening. Some wanted more time to share the warm feelings generated by the Von Newman massage.

We suggest that people giving a body party balance structure and freedom a little more carefully than we did. At future parties, we would select only one or two games, just enough to create the right mood.

The Conceal-Reveal and To-Strip-or-not-to-Strip games tend to leave people relaxed and comfortable, ready to open up to each other verbally. The Tom Jones dinner and the fashion show tend to turn adults into playful children who want to dance, joke, or get into mischief. The Von Newman massage makes people mellow, and leaves them quiet and misty eyed.

Giving a successful body party takes no special training, only a willingness to take the lead in introducing your friends to something new. We believe you can have the same sort of body joy and interpersonal closeness at your body-joy party that we had at ours. With or without nudity, you provide an atmosphere where people are encouraged to do what makes their bodies comfortable and what makes them feel comfortable about their bodies. We'll now suggest some body-party activities that enable people to be seen, listened to, and touched in loving and enjoyable ways.

ACTIVITIES FOR "CLOTHING-ON" AND CLOTHING-OPTIONAL BODY PARTIES

Body parties won't just happen; you need to take some responsibility—to plan, nudge, coax, explain. The main goals are informality and body comfort. Introduce foods that are simple, old-fashioned, natural. Experiment with sitting on floor cushions instead of chairs, using your fingers instead of silverware, finger-tip towels instead of linen or paper napkins.

Facials

As with a clothing-optional party, your invitations should let your guests know what to expect. We used the following invitation for one of our clothing-on parties that featured the giving of facials.

TIRED OF THE ORDINARY?
WANT SOMETHING DIFFERENT?
JOIN EMILY AND BETTY FOR A BODY PARTY

Date: July 10, 1976

Time: 2:00-8:00 P.M.

What to Expect: Facials—given with affection and guaranteed to make you look and feel better than ever.

Fun—join us in some new ways to play.

Food—A light supper about 6:00 P.M.

If the idea of a party to give facials seems bizarre, remember that our faces rarely get touched by human hands other than our own. If you doubt this, try to remember the last time someone, other than a sex partner, touched your face in a loving manner, or the last time you touched another person's face just as a gesture of affection. Allowing someone to give us a facial helps us accept our faces as they are. The flaws, blemishes, and wrinkles become less important as loving ministrations tell us that no matter how we look we are lovable. Giving a facial also allows you to express your tender feelings; if you aren't feeling tender to begin with, caring for another person's exposed and vulnerable face can make you feel that way.

Dancing

One friend of ours selects a wide variety of music—jazz, rock, soul, classical, marching, romantic, folk—and has guests dance alone to each type of music according to the mood it brings out in him, first with eyes closed and then open. She varies the music, and the guests are not aware just when there will be a change of pace.

Mirror dancing is great for helping strangers get acquainted. Partners face one another and, keeping time with the music, move as if dancing alone in front of a mirror, taking turns being the dancer-leader and the mirror-follower.

Exercises

You and your friends can share your favorite exercises with one another. We gave such a party once. Ask each guest to demonstrate his favorite exercise or series of exercises and tell its benefits—stretching, reducing, toning, relaxing, etc. Then everybody does it together, with musical accompaniment, with the person who suggested it leading and helping the others to get it right. Types of exercises can include some yoga, tai chi, ballet exercises, traditional calisthenics, isometrics.

The Body-Compliment Game

This is an activity that will promote affectionate touching as well as encourage your guests to look at each other's bodies openly and freely, focusing on positive aspects. Participants form a circle, all sitting. One person then stands up, looks at the person to his left and says something nice about his body. It is very important to make eye contact and to use the person's name and the phrase, "I like your _____." He might say something like, "Larry, I like your muscular arms," or "Thelma, I like your bellybutton." The person he speaks to then stands up and responds by saying, "Thank you. And I like my _____." He then turns to the next person and offers a compliment. After everyone has a turn, go around the circle again in the opposite direction so that everyone has an opportunity to receive a body compliment from those on both sides of him.

Strip Bean Bag

Participants stand in a circle and while music is being played, throw a bean bag or a sofa pillow to one another. Like musical chairs, the music is stopped every now and then (by a nonplaying guest) at unexpected intervals. The one who has the bean bag when the music stops must take off something he is wearing and put it in the middle of the circle. (At a clothes-on party, people have many things they can remove without embarrassment—jewelry, belts, shoes, etc.—and the guests can drop out when they've removed as much as they are comfortable with.) A time limit is set and at the end of the game, participants are permitted to put their clothes back on, take more clothes off, or try on one another's clothes. This game is even more fun than strip poker for it goes faster, and group members can gang up on a willing and extroverted participant by throwing him the pillow frequently so he'll be forced to take off more clothes than anyone else.

Nude Man's Bluff

This game can be played in a living room, backyard, or swimming pool. Participants gather around one person who is blindfolded. Each person in turn presents a part of his or her anatomy—an arm, leg, toe, elbow, ear, nose, etc.—to the blindfolded person, carefully guiding his hand so that he can touch that part and no other. The blindfolded person then tries to guess who he is touching. When he guesses correctly, the person who has been caught has a turn being blindfolded.

The "Move Like I Move" Game

Guests stand up and form a circle. One person stands in the center and moves or wiggles some body parts in a simple rhythmic way, over and over. When he gets his movements down pat so that others can readily mimic him, he beckons to someone in the circle to join him in the center and they do it together and all the other people do it also. After his partner has gotten the movement and rhythm down pat, the original leader points his finger at his partner who starts a new movement. The former leader goes back into the circle and the whole process is repeated. We defy you to try playing this game with a straight face.

Water Fun: the Hot Tub

The opportunity to use water facilities in body-liberating ways is almost unlimited, particularly if the facilities are secluded enough to permit nudity. With water, nudity becomes a natural part of the activities. After all, few activities are more pleasurable than "skinny dipping."

The whirlpool bath (often called a Jacuzzi, the brand name of the most popular manufacturer) encourages socializing while bathing and encourages new attitudes toward bodies and nudity. Though originally used as a therapeutic device for orthopedic and arthritic patients, whirlpool baths are now being used by many people for relaxing and socializing activities. One couple we know even has one in the living room, which can be opened to the sky via a skylight, and when they entertain, instead of an after-dinner brandy, they turn on the jets and have an after-dinner bath.

"Hot-tubbing" originated in Santa Barbara, California, when someone got hold of one of those redwood vats used for making wine, rigged up an old heater, and filled the vat with hot water and good friends. The news about the pleasures of hot-tubbing in water up to 115° or 120° has spread all over the country. A hot tub is cheaper than a swimming pool but also smaller and more limited in use. A five-foot tub holds about eight people, while a six-footer holds thirteen—if they are friendly and willing to snuggle. Hot tubs truly make solitary bathing seem like a sin. It might be possible to be uptight when stepping into a hot tub, but it is almost impossible to be so when stepping out.

Water Fun: The Floating Technique

This technique, patterned after one originally used in Paul Bindrim's marathons (see Chapter 5), has become a very popular one in many nude workshops. However, you don't need to be in a workshop to learn how to do this nor do you need a person with experience to show you how. In this procedure the person who is "floated," preferably in warm water, gets the feeling that other people can and will take care of him even if he lies back and does nothing. He senses that people can be trusted to be gentle toward him. One or more (ideally four or five) persons stand around a volunteer who floats on his back. One puts a hand under his head. Others support his body in various places while they gently move him around in the water, occasionally stroking all parts of his body. All of this is done without any talking. After a while one person gathers the volunteer in his arms like a baby and goes to the pool steps or the side of the pool and holds him in a rocking position, stroking his forehead and hair.

It is necessary to take the experience seriously and not splash, tickle, or joke when floating someone. Remember, when a person allows you to float him, he is showing that he trusts you by giving you the honor and responsibility of taking care of his body. Be sure his head doesn't go under, that water isn't splashed in his face, and that when he is stroked, it is with the intention of showing him affection.

Massage

As you and your friends become increasingly comfortable with your bodies, you might like to give a massage body-party. However, you must be extremely careful in the way you invite people and how you structure this particular party because to many people the word "massage" has sexual connotations. Massage must be presented for what it can be—a rare opportunity to get to know another person through touch and to show affection by relieving body tensions.

Massage can be sensual, nurturing, vigorous, energizing, mystical, sexual, depending on the kind of movements you use. One person can massage another—all over or just certain places where tension tends to build up, such as in the back, neck, and legs. Or several people can cooperate and give one person a massage. (We gave you directions for one form of group massage, the "Von Newman," earlier in the chapter.)

Concern over getting a sexy feeling keeps many people from seeking a massage or from enjoying it fully when they have one. What they don't realize is that the amount of sexual charge built up during a massage depends on the attitude of the person giving it, the way it is given, and the expectations of the person getting massaged.

William Mueller, mentioned previously, trains his students to minimize sexual implications of a massage and show recognition of a person's individuality and humanness. Here are some of his suggestions.

The person giving the massage should picture himself as a parent and the person receiving the massage as a child. Imagining these roles sets up a mental attitude of "I am going to take care of you now; you can relax and feel safe with me." You become a nurturing friend, not a potential sex partner, and your thoughts are conveyed by your touch.

The following are some of Mueller's techniques:

When massaging up the leg toward the thigh, keep your hands on the outside of the legs. Thus your hand is going not toward the genitals, but toward the hip. When you do the inside of the leg, move your hands toward the person's feet. Any movement going directly toward his genitals makes a person wonder what will happen next.

With the same principle in mind, when working on the stomach, start above the pubic hair line and go up toward the chest and neck instead of moving the hand downward toward the genitals. When moving from the neck to the stomach, move your hands along the side of the body toward the hips.

Pressure and speed help determine the mood conveyed by touch. Movements that are light and quick and playful—that stimulate the surface of the skin—are generally more sexual than heavier pressure that concentrates on the underlying tissue. When the movement is slower and heavier, when the whole hand is used rather than just the fingers, the touch is more nurturing. Be sure to use a firm, steady pressure to move over the breasts, not a light, teasing touch.

Your touch will frequently tell the person you are massaging more about what you are feeling than words can. If you and he are feeling comfortable and relaxed, silence can enhance the massage. On the other hand, if you are uncomfortable for some reason, that discomfort may be communicated to the person you are massaging. If this occurs, tell him of your concerns. Sharing your feelings in this way will keep you from making the person you are massaging feel uncomfortable.

At this point you may not be convinced that either you or your friends would ever feel free enough to participate in body parties or in any kind of social nudity. It may seem to you that the activities we have described will always be limited to a very small segment of the population. We disagree. We believe that within five years the type of participatory nudity we have been describing will be commonplace. In the next chapter we'll take a look at some pioneers in the area of body liberation who are helping to change attitudes—and laws—that have inhibited or prohibited the widespread acceptance of social nudity.

Chapter 15
The Politics
of Going Bare

> Some people in authority have the idea it isn't worthwhile to learn to enjoy yourself and that anybody who wants to is in some way evil. The time has come for us to develop sensible attitudes toward pleasure, to become *responsible* hedonists. As it is now people either unthinkingly deny themselves or equally unthinkingly indulge themselves.
>
> Ed Lange,
> Director, Elysium Fields

One hot day in August 1970, Chad Merrill Smith, a young Californian, and a male friend went to the beach. Finding the area deserted, Smith took off his clothes, stretched out on the sand, and fell asleep. In the interim, several people came to the beach, and some complained to a policeman about Smith's nudity. He woke up to find himself under arrest for violating Section 314 of the California Penal Code, which states, "Every person who willfully and lewdly ... exposes his person, or the private parts thereof, in any public place, or in any place where there are present other persons to be offended or annoyed thereby ... is guilty of a misdemeanor."

The word "misdemeanor" suggests a mild penalty. But Smith's penalty for being found guilty of indecent exposure was a much harsher one than that given to people found guilty of violating other misdemeanor laws—because the consequences will affect him for the rest of his life.

Under arrest—and before conviction—a suspect's fingerprints and description are filed with the State Bureau of Criminal Identification and Investigation. If the person is convicted, additional information, including his photograph, is forwarded to the same state bureau, and the person must register as a sex offender with the chief of police in the city in which he lives. From then on, every time he moves, he must be sure to file a notification of his change of address within ten days.

These penalties, designed for true sex offenders, become oppressive and unjust when applied to someone caught innocently sunbathing in the nude on an isolated public beach.

Smith decided to challenge the interpretation that just being naked constituted lewdness. Nearly two years after his arrest, on June 13, 1972, the California Supreme Court, in a highly significant and body-liberating decision, ruled that the naked body is not "inherently" obscene. "Mere nudity," said the court "does not constitute a form of sexual 'activity'." Thus Smith, who sunbathed nude without intentionally directing attention to his genitals for sexual purposes, did not "lewdly" expose his private parts within the meaning of the indecent exposure statute.

The significance of the Smith decision is that there is now no legal prohibition against mere nudity in public in California—unless a city or county wants to outlaw it. Even then, a person arrested for nudity is charged only with violating that ordinance and usually only has to pay a small fine; he no longer needs to fear a lifetime of harassment as a suspected sex offender. As people in other states begin challenging "indecent exposure" laws in cases involving mere nudity, the Smith decision is likely to serve as a precedent.

Smith was the forerunner of a trend that reached massive proportions in California in the early 1970s—the trend toward sunbathing and swimming in the nude at California beaches. Although clandestine skinny-dipping at isolated beaches has always occurred, the nude-beach movement in the United States probably "officially" began about 1967 at San Gregorio Beach near San Francisco. By 1974, as many as two thousand nude sunbathers might be found on just one beach, such as the popular Brooks Beach at Venice, within the Los Angeles city limits.

Stymied by the Smith decision, the police and sheriff's department in Los Angeles began trying to fight beach nudity by other means, such as arresting people for disturbing the peace or trespassing on private property, even though in some cases (such as Pirate's Cove near Malibu) the public had been using the private beaches without protest from the owners for many years. The authorities' efforts were encouraged by beach property owners who worried about property values and by small groups of conservative citizens who saw nude bathing as evidence of moral decay. In one incident at Pirate's Cove, in August 1972, twenty-five deputies in five squad cars, a paddy wagon, and a helicopter descended on the crowded beach and hauled away—in handcuffs—six people who had been peacefully enjoying the sun. No one was convicted of trespassing, however. The defendants were offered a deal; if they paid court costs of twenty-five dollars, their cases would be dismissed. The one defendant who refused this plea bargaining had his case dismissed for lack of evidence.

The growing popularity of beach nudity attracted sensational media coverage, which in turn attracted thousands of clothed sight-seers. Pressured by conservative taxpayers, in July 1974, the Los Angeles City Council passed an ordinance banning nudity on all Los Angeles beaches.

BEACHFRONT U.S.A.

Upset by official intimidation and harassment, and believing nude sunbathing and swimming to be a constitutional right—part of the freedom of expression protected by the First Amendment—German-born Eugene Callen, a Santa Monica engineer who had witnessed the raid on Pirate's Cove, formed an organization called Beachfront U.S.A. for the protection of nude beaches. Although he points out that in Europe nude beaches are commonplace and that he believes bathing suits are an obsolete remnant of Victorian morality, Callen does not consider himself a nudist. He objects to the implication that there are two kinds of people, nudists and non-nudists. Callen simply wants to bring about what he calls natural or rational bathing in the nations' water areas, both publicly and privately owned: "It's not a matter of dogma. I believe that someday nude bathing will be extended to motels and apartment buildings. In Germany and other cities in Europe, a number of municipal swimming pools now have nude bathing on certain nights. In time this will happen here."

Beachfront U.S.A. issued a "Free Beach Manifesto," which made the following points:

1. Nudity on the beach is neither lewd nor indecent.
2. A growing number of young Americans, currently comprising several millions, want to establish nude beaches on public and private lands.
3. Democratic principles clearly imply that local governments have the obligation to implement these legitimate demands by officially designating some beach areas for nude bathing.
4. The number and extent of these areas should be proportional to the percentage of persons who indicate a preference for nude beaches.

Beachfront has fought for nude beaches on four fronts: (1) It has challenged (unsuccessfully) the constitutionality of the Los Angeles city ordinance banning nude bathing; (2) It has pressured Los Angeles County officials into promising to establish a nude beach, although it now feels the county reneged on this promise; (3) It got the Sheriff's office to unofficially agree not to prosecute nude bathers at Pirate's Cove, despite the fact that Los Angeles County passed an anti-nudity ordinance in July 1975; (4) It has concentrated on informing the public about what is really going on in the free beach fight and toward changing people's attitudes regarding nudity.

Beachfront has been working with organizations in other parts of the country to establish free beaches. One joint effort was Nude Beach Day, held August 8, 1976, when free-beach supporters flocked to beaches all over the country to indicate to authorities by their numbers that they be heeded. One of the larger rallies was held at Zuma Beach in Los Angeles County, where two thousand people showed up. Even though the demonstrators were clothed, the police were present in force with squad cars, helicopters, and on horseback. Such demonstrations bring to mind earlier protests in which demonstrators *have* taken off their clothes for a cause (Lady Godiva's nude ride to protest her husband's unfair taxation of the peasants; St. Francis of Assisi walking naked through the streets when his bishop rebuked him).

The future of nude beaches depend on how many people see them as an idea whose time has come. Dr. Alex Comfort, author of *The Joy of Sex*, believes opposition comes from a small (though vocal) minority. Writing in the Introduction to Leon Elder's *Free Beaches*, Comfort says:

> "... Nudity—or rather, nonfuss about concealing the human body—is becoming more generally accepted. If people with drip-dry skins still swim dressed, however skimpily, it is because of pressure from the fringe of public morality. Normal America, like normal Scandinavia, is becoming not ideologically nudist, but simply fussless."

THE BATTLE FOR PARTICIPATORY NUDITY

Another battle being waged for the right of people to enjoy going bare—in this case for educational purposes—is being led by Ed Lange, founder of Elysium Institute and Director of Elysium Field, the clothing-optional growth center in Topanga Canyon.

A successful professional photographer and a long-time participant in the American Sunbathing Association and the Western Sunbathing Association, Lange became dissatisfied with the early nudist publications and decided to create one that would depict the human form in a more honest and natural manner. In 1959 he created *Eden*, a nudist magazine, and in 1961 he established Elysium, Inc., his own publishing firm which has produced films, magazines, and books aimed at educating the public about the human body.

Lange's pictures are sensual, lively, human, and unairbrushed. Because of his belief that "the public must be allowed to see for themselves through pictures and text that man unclothed is a magnificent being," Lange found himself in the early 1960s in conflict with postal authorities who equated nudity with obscenity. But by 1963 he had won that battle and became the first publisher of unretouched nudist magazines to obtain second-class mailing privileges with the Post Office.

Lange's real battle with the powers-that-be began when he opened Elysium Field as a place that, unlike traditional nudist resorts and growth centers, offered people, nude if they chose to be, an opportunity to do a lot of inner searching and to learn about their bodies, feelings, and sexuality. But Los Angeles County had, in 1939, enacted an anti-nudity ordinance so strict that it made even the nudity of three members of the same family illegal if one of them was of the opposite sex. Elysium Field was automatically in violation of this law. Lange was charged and tried. But during his trial he challenged the constitutionality of the ordinance, and won.

In 1970 the Los Angeles County Board of Supervisors enacted another ordinance. This one required places permitting nudity to acquire a license—and one of the supervisors stated openly that the purpose of the ordinance was to enable the county to deny the license to certain nudist places. This ordinance was also found unconstitutional.

The third time Lange was hauled before the authorities was in 1975, and this time it was the county regional planning commission. Some irate neighbors tried to have him and Elysium declared a public nuisance. But because Lange was able to prove that there were no loud noises coming from Elysium (radios, televisions, and public address systems are not permitted), that neighbors could not see the nudity (the place is enclosed by fences and much shrubbery), and that the number of cars permitted in the parking lot had not been excessive (which had been one of the alleged offenses), he was able to rebut the complaints.

Although as this book goes to press there is yet a fourth challenge—on the grounds of violating a new zoning law—one enacted years after Elysium began. However, Elysium continues to flourish. Whenever attack brings the growth center to the attention of television and newspapers, new applications for admission roll in. It is currently supported by one thousand adults and four hundred children, and many others attend the weekend seminars. Other growth centers modeled along the same lines are being planned in other areas, and Lange doesn't think they can be stopped.

RELIGIOUS ATTITUDES

Robert Cromey, an Episcopalian minister for fourteen years, still in good standing in his diocese, left his fulltime ministry for a private psychotherapy practice in San Francisco. Cromey wanted to work with *whole* people—those with bodies and feelings as well as with minds and souls—something he could not do within his church, which takes, he believes, a strictly intellectual approach to religious experience.

According to him, there is no official Episcopal view on nudity: "There is nothing in its formularies as to whether nudity is good or bad, right or wrong—or anything. The only time something is wrong is when you do it, then someone will say it is wrong for some reason." Cromey, who believes that nudity helps people be more honest and straightforward, wishes the churches would provide more opportunities—including perhaps the use of nude workshops—for people to become more open with themselves and others.

He points out how frequently and reverently the word *body* is used in the Christian religion—the body of Christ, the body of the church, the body of Christian people. But, says Cromey, the church itself has, in a sense, been disembodied and it needs to be rejoined with its body—to deal with the emotional and physical side of existence as well as with the intellectual and spiritual.

OUTLOOK FOR THE FUTURE

What does the future hold for those who believe the right to go bare is a basic one? Noted civil liberties lawyer Stanley Fleishman, who defended Elysium's right to stay in business, believes that the right of an individual to be nude has First Amendment overtones and is part of his fundamental right to privacy, which the state cannot interfere with except for compelling reasons. According to Fleishman, the laws on nudity are in a state of flux—there is a fair amount of law developing which supports the right of public nudity and also a fair amount going the other way. Fleishman believes that, in time, the view favoring some forms of public nudity will be adopted into law.

We hope further that the day is coming when the human body in its entirety will no longer be taboo. When that day comes, there will be no need for a book on body liberation. In fact, much of the time and energy now spent compulsively keeping bodies covered or trying to change them into something they can never be will be spent instead on more important things—such as building political and educational systems that develop loving human beings, cleaning the air and keeping it clean, writing sonnets and symphonies, lying on the grass contemplating the universe or one's own life, and celebrating the human body as Walt Whitman did, in his poetry.

Although Whitman lived in the Victorian era, he was able to see beyond the body prejudices of his age and become the poet laureate of body liberation. His essay, "A Sun-Bath—Nakedness," written in 1878, expresses his belief in the *need* in all of us to be sometimes naked if we are to be liberated.

> Nature was naked, and I was also. It was too lazy, soothing, and joyous—equable to speculate about. Yet I might have thought somehow in this vein: Perhaps the inner never-lost rapport we hold with earth, light, air, trees, etc., is not to be realized through eyes and mind only, but through the whole corporeal body, which I will not have blinded or bandaged any more than the eyes. Sweet, sane, still Nakedness in Nature!—Ah, if poor, sick, prurient humanity in cities might really know you once more! Is not nakedness then indecent? No, not inherently. It is your thought, your sophistication, your fear, your respectability, that is indecent.

Epilogue: Declaration of Body Independence

While we were working on this book, we began to fantasize about what might happen if the principles of body liberation became widely accepted. One of our fantasies was particularly beautiful to us—the idea of a Body Independence Day to be celebrated once a year. And just as during our national independence celebration we celebrate our liberation from the political tyranny of Great Britain, during our imaginary Body Independence Day people would celebrate their liberation from the tyranny of negative body attitudes.

We thought an appropriate day to celebrate Body Independence would be on March 24—Wilhelm Reich's birthday—because in many ways he was the father of body liberation. In addition, our celebration of the rebirth of the human body would take place only three days after the official beginning of spring, when nature itself experiences a rebirth.

We drew up a Declaration of Body Independence that might serve as a symbol of people's determination to gain and retain their natural birthright—*their body freedom*. We used as our model, of course, that inspiring document symbolizing our national determination to be free as a nation and as individuals. Here is our version:

Declaration of Body Independence

When in the course of human events, it becomes necessary for a people to dissolve the customs, laws, and beliefs that have kept them from being connected with their bodies and to assert their right to liberate their bodies in the manner which the laws of nature and nature's God have intended, a decent respect to the opinions of mankind requires that they should declare these causes which impel them to the separation.

We hold these truths to be self-evident—that all bodies are created equal, not equal in looks and inherent abilities, but equally worthwhile in the eyes of God, the law, and other men; that our bodies are endowed by our Creator with certain unalienable rights, that among these are the right of our bodies to sufficient physical, emotional, and intellectual nourishment to develop to their full potential; the right of our bodies to discover and follow their own destiny without being told by any other body—be it the state, a corporation, or a mate—when to work, play, make love, or die; and the right of our bodies to experience pleasure.

We also believe that when any customs, laws, or beliefs, instituted among men, become destructive of these body rights it is the obligation of the people to alter or abolish them. Such customs, laws, and beliefs, long established, shall not be cast off lightly but when they seem about to create an absolute despotism, it is our right, it is our duty, to get rid of them. The history of the body abuses to which we have been subjected for centuries is a history of repeated injuries and usurpations all having as their object the establishment of an absolute tyranny over our bodies. To prove this, let facts be submitted to a candid world.

>Body tyrants have divided us by letting us believe that the color of some bodies is superior to the color of other bodies and that young bodies are superior to old bodies.
>
>Body tyrants have blinded us to the awesome beauty of the human body by making us afraid to look at and proudly acknowledge our *entire* naked bodies.
>
>Body tyrants have starved us for comforting and loving human touch by limiting the number of others we are allowed to touch and by cruelly rationing the occasions on which we may touch.
>
>Body tyrants have robbed us of our full and joyous humanity by tricking us into believing our bodies are like machines and that, like machines, they are only valuable for what they can do.
>
>Body tyrants have cheated us of the opportunity to explore the untapped potential of our bodies by teaching us our bodies aren't worth studying.

Body tyrants have imprisoned our tears and anger and grief within our bodies by telling us that some emotions are not acceptable.

Body tyrants have deafened us so that we can no longer listen to the wisdom of our own bodies but instead hear their incessant demands on our bodies—eat now, defecate now, create now, play now, make love now, die now.

We, therefore, solemnly publish and declare that our bodies are, and ought to be, free and independent entities and that all connections with the body tyrants of the past are, and ought to be, totally dissolved. As free and independent bodies we each have the full power and right—but not the obligation—to seek body liberation. And to make the principles stated in this declaration a reality, we do mutually pledge to each other all of the aid and support we can give for this purpose.

After writing our Declaration of Body Independence we learned we aren't the only ones with such a dream. Some people in Minneapolis, who have already set up a foundation called the Body Freedom Foundation, declared July 4, 1977, the first annual Independence Day. They invited people on that day to "appear without clothing, each at an appropriate place, by their own standards, and the clothing taboo will be broken." (The address of the committee is in our list of addresses in the back of the book.)

So we thought it appropriate to end this book with our support of the idea of an annual, nationwide Body Independence Day. No matter on what day it is celebrated or how it is celebrated, it seems clear that the widespread acceptance of the principles of body liberation is not fantasy but a vision shared by many people.

BODY INDEPENDENCE DAY, 1997—
THE AUTHORS' VISION

Fifteen-year-old Marcie Anderson woke up early with that special feeling of anticipation she always got on holidays. It was March 24, 1997, Body Independence Day. This would be the fifth such annual holiday that Marcie—and the rest of the nation—had celebrated. Already the day had acquired its own special set of holiday traditions. There was going to be a big celebration at the community center in the park. (Since March was such an unpredictable month, weatherwise, the celebration was always planned for inside—with the understanding that it would be moved outdoors in good weather.) On this particular March day, it was as though nature wanted to cooperate—the sun was shining through a cloudless sky.

Marcie hurried downstairs where she joined the rest of the family—her mother, father, grandparents, two older brothers, and eight-month-old sister. This was the part of the day Marcie especially looked forward to—the time the family reviewed old, and drew up new, "body contracts." Every year on this date families all over the nation made such contracts with each other.

The Anderson family kept their body contracts in a special folder. As they are pulled out and reviewed, there is a lot of bragging (when they have been lived up to) and rationalizing (when they haven't). Marcie, who has a tendency to overweight, had pledged to give her body the pleasure of moving more freely *minus* fifteen pounds and the family now demanded a "weigh-in." Marcie has not only lived up to her contract, but signed another to give her new body yoga lessons once a week. She also extended the second part of her contract—to rub her mother's back twice a week—for another year.

After the signing of the new contracts, the family did a series of exercises together—not rigorous calisthenics—but exercises that allow them to move and stretch their bodies in new and graceful ways. Then they shared a breakfast that was both nutritious and delicious. The exercise and breakfast routine was not limited to Body Independence Day in the Anderson family; the family had instituted them as a once-a-week part of the family routine two Body Independence Days ago.

The family does have one ritual that had become associated with Body Independence Day—a family bath. The Anderson house had been remodeled so that the toilet facilities were separate from the bathing facilities. The bathroom was just that—a *bath* room. In the center of the room was a large round tub big enough for six to eight people. This tub—which would have had to be custom-built only twenty years earlier—was purchased from the Sears Catalog at a very reasonable price. The room also included a shower so that family members could wash off before joining the others in the warm water. Although members of the family frequently bathed together, it wasn't often that the entire family had a chance to share this pleasurable experience.

Bath time was the very favorite experience of Marcie's baby sister who—held securely in her brother's arms—splashed happily in the tub. After the bath, Marcie's mother wrapped her baby (naked except for diapers) next to her own naked torso in a specially designed shawl—similar to that worn by Balinese mothers. The shawl let her move her body and arms freely yet it held the baby securely next to her and gave both of them skin contact.

After preparing a picnic lunch, the family went over to the park to celebrate the holiday with their neighbors. Marcie joined several of her school friends and the group of boys and girls linked arms, held hands, put their arms around each other's shoulders and otherwise casually touched each other's bodies.

The crowd quieted down as the mayor stepped to the podium and read the Declaration of Body Independence. Marcie listened intently as he read.

After the reading, the mayor talked a little about the history of Body Independence Day. Although Marcie had learned some of this in her high school social studies class, she never tired of hearing how it got started:

In the late 1970s, shortly before the anniversary of Wilhelm Reich's birthday, television and radio studios and newspapers all over the country received a copy of a very unusual press release. This press release announced the first annual Body Independence Day, and included a copy of the Declaration of Body Independence.

Some of the announcers at the television and radio studios read the release (adding joking commentary) and some of the newspapers printed the press release verbatim. Surprisingly, the idea—presented as a crackpot news item by the media—began to catch on with the public. The group responsible for the press release began lecturing, appearing on television talk shows, and writing articles. They were not crackpots, but people from every walk of life and profession who had seen no hope for social reform until people learned to like their own bodies. They repeated over and over that only when we have a nation of self-loving people will we be able to truly love others and to take the steps necessary for a better way of life.

The body liberation movement progressed in much the same way that most other social reform movements have progressed in this country. Jokes about "clothes-shedding body libbers" replaced jokes about "bra-burning women's libbers." Then came repression from the authorities. For the first few years bathers participating in mass nude-ins were sometimes arrested with a great deal of "overkill," and pictures of naked, peaceful bathers being hauled away in handcuffs by armed policemen are now historical curiosities. But soon there were minor legal victories, and then, in 1985, the Supreme Court in a historic decision declared that the right to be nude was part of the right of privacy and the freedom of expression guaranteed by the First Amendment. This decision was followed by one in 1987 that declared all state tax-supported recreational facilities must provide "equal facilities or time" for nudists under the equal protection clause of the fourteenth amendment—and the major battle was won.

The impact of that law went far beyond the public campgrounds, beaches, parks, swimming pools, lakes, and rivers that now had special clothing-optional areas for those interested in nude bathing, sunbathing, picnicking, and camping. Hotels and motels—under the interstate commerce clause of the constitution—also had to provide clothing-optional hours for their guests at swimming pools, saunas, and jacuzzis. Private recreational areas found they could not compete successfully unless they met the demand for clothing-optional facilities. Most private apartment houses began posting times when people could swim or jacuzzi nude—and some openly catered to people interested in a clothing-optional lifestyle.

Businesses discovered they could make a profit from this new American attitude toward the human body. Designers were able to introduce new styles of clothing—outfits that were easily slipped on and off whenever convenient. This clothing was frequently designed to be worn by either sex and was flowing and sensuous—freeing the body instead of restricting it.

Furniture, cars, buildings, homes—all the accoutrements of a technological society—were designed with *people* in mind (taking into account the shape and functions of their bodies). There were more things designed for people's pleasure—massage equipment, new types of pools and jacuzzis, games—and fewer things designed to appeal to their destructive or competitive side—war games, guns, high-powered cars.

While a lot of what the mayor was saying was ancient history to Marcie, she could remember the fuss in the community when the body liberation movement spilled over into the public school system. Although government funds were being used to sponsor brief announcements on television about bodies—one-minute messages about the principles of body liberation—the leaders in the movement felt it could not completely succeed until children absorbed these new body attitudes as a routine part of their education.

When the principal of the local elementary school, instead of punishing misbehaving students, sent them to a special "frustration room" where they could work off their emotional frustration by punching pillows and screaming freely, the PTA marched in protest. When the principal of the junior high school added to the curriculum an excellent workshop on body education the PTA again marched in protest—but in vain. And last year when the high school swimming pool was made clothing-optional two nights a week, the PTA marched—right into the pool where they swam nude.

After the mayor completed his speech there was a special pageant in honor of the 100th anniversary of Wilhelm Reich's birthday. This pageant depicted the naked human body in all its glory and in all its stages from infancy to old age—showing the beauty in each and every stage. Then the crowd began to wander through the exhibits. There were slide shows, tables with books about the body, and many, many films. There were films on non-drug methods for treating bodily discomfort and preventing bodily disease, films on topics such as reflexology and acupressure massage, on non-stress methods of learning, such as suggestology, on consciousness-raising methods, on love-making techniques. The times and places for free city-sponsored classes on all aspects of body liberation were posted and a consultant was available to offer suggestions as to which classes would be most suitable for particular individuals.

There were also numerous two-hour workshops that allowed people to experience something good for the body—the latest massage techniques, biofeedback equipment, emotional release techniques, dance therapy, "centering" methods such as meditation—and all were free to the public.

In addition, there were classes on nutrition, on fasting, on stretching, toning, and relaxing exercises. There were special classes for photographers which featured nude models of all ages and both sexes. In the workshops and all of the recreational facilities at the park the wearing of many, few, or no clothes at all was permitted.

It was a full day. Marcie's small body was bone tired, but it was a good kind of tiredness—a happy kind. She was silent and thoughtful as she rode home from the park in her parents' car. When her dad asked the reason for her silence, she snuggled up to him and said, "I've been wondering about how people in the past could have really believed all those things about bodies. Imagine having to wear a suit to go swimming. Imagine not being able to touch someone just because they were the same sex as you. Imagine being ashamed of your body. I guess they just didn't know any better."

Appendix: Where to Go for More Information

NUDE BEACHES, RESORTS, AND TOURS

By writing to these addresses, you can find out where the existing legal clothing-optional or nudist places are located, what is going on in the fight to legalize clothing-optional beaches, and ways you can get involved.

American Sunbathing Association, Inc.
810 North Mills Avenue
Orlando, Florida 32803
(Information on nude resorts.)

Associated Students—Campus Activities
University of California
Santa Cruz, California 95060
(Information on nude beach movement in northern California.)

Bare in Mind
PO Box 111
Colton, California 92324
(Five dollars for a one-year subscription to the only independent nudist newspaper in United States.)

Beachfront U.S.A.
PO Box 90191
Los Angeles, California 90009
(Information on nude beach movement in southern California.)

Free the Free Beach
PO Box 300
Truro, Cape Cod, Massachusetts 02666
(For information on the nude beach movement in New England area, send a stamped, self-addressed envelope.)

Free Beaches
PO Box 132
Oshkosh, Wisconsin 54901
(Send Free Beaches a stamped, self-addressed envelope. They'll send you the latest information on the nude beach movement throughout the country.)

Nude Beaches Committee
PO Box 99581
San Diego, California 92109
(Include a stamped, self-addressed envelope for information on the nude beach movement in the San Diego area.)

Sun Coral
2-43 University Center
800 North State College Boulevard
Fullerton, California 92634
(A group of college students fighting for the legalization of clothing-optional areas.)

Elysium Tours (no connection with Elysium Field)
1701 Clinton Street
Suite 207
Los Angeles, California 90026

Skinny Dip Tours
30 East 42nd Street
New York, New York

V.I.B. Tours (Vacations in the Buff)
244 East 46th Street
New York, New York 10017
(Information on travel to clothing-optional areas abroad.)

GROWTH CENTERS AND EDUCATIONAL INSTITUTIONS

Write these places for the latest information on new trends in the human potential movement (including nude workshops and therapy) and lists of growth centers across the nation.

Association for Humanistic Psychology
325 Ninth Street
San Francisco, California 94103

(Send a stamped, self-addressed envelope for a list of growth centers across the nation or a list of colleges with humanistically orientated programs.)

Elysium Field
814 Robinson Road
Topanga, California 90290
(Clothing-optional growth center. Send a stamped, self-addressed envelope for information.)

Elysium: a Journal of the Senses
Elysium Growth Press
5436 Fernwood Avenue
Los Angeles, California 90027
(Two dollars for a one-year subscription—four issues. One dollar for single copy. Includes information about latest trends in the human potential movement.)

Center for Marital and Sexual Studies
5199 East Pacific Coast Highway
Long Beach, California 90804
(This is a training center for sex therapists from all over the nation as well as a clinic for sexual therapy. Send a stamped, self-addressed envelope for further information.)

Esalen Institute
Big Sur, California 93920
(Please include stamped, self-addressed envelope.)

Man-Woman Institute
PO Box 15026
Long Beach, California 90815
(Send a stamped, self-addressed envelope for workshops, vacation trips, and other events—clothing on and clothing optional—offered by Emily Coleman.)

Sandstone
21400 Saddle Peak Road
Topanga, California 90290

The National Center for the Exploration of Human Potential
976 Chalcedony Street
San Diego, California 92109
(Please include a stamped, self-addressed envelope.)

BODY-LIBERATING THERAPIES

Write these addresses for information on the type of therapy you are interested in and where you can obtain a therapist.

The Alexander Technique

The American Center for the Alexander Technique, Inc. has offices at the following locations:

811 23rd Street
Santa Monica, California 90403
c/o Judith Stransky, Director

931 Elizabeth Street
San Francisco, California 94114
c/o Frank Ottiwell, Director

142 West End Avenue
New York, New York 10023
c/o Judith Leibowitz, Director

Bioenergetics

Institute for Bioenergetic Analysis
71 Park Avenue
New York, New York 10016

Feldenkrais

Feldenkrais Method
811 23rd Street
Santa Monica, California 90403
c/o Judith Stransky

Medical Orgonomy

Elsworth F. Baker
Orgonomic Publications, Inc.
PO Box 565
Ansonia Station
New York, New York 10023

Radix

Radix Institute
PO Box 3218
Santa Monica, California 90403

Rolfing and Structural Patterning

Rolf Institute
PO Box 1868
Boulder, Colorado 80302

HOLISTIC HEALTH CENTERS AND ORGANIZATIONS

Write these addresses for information on holistic health centers, practitioners, or reading material. Although most of the centers are located in California, some of them may be able to help you locate people interested in the concept of holistic health in your area.

Association for Holistic Health
Box 23231
San Diego, California 92123
(The Association is bringing together individuals and organizations dedicated to providing centers, education, and research in holistic health.)

Center for the Healing Arts
11081 Missouri Avenue
Los Angeles, California 90025
(The Center for the Healing Arts is an independent, non-profit organization dedicated to exploring the multi-dimensional nature of healing and health maintenance through seminars and workshops, research programs, consultation services, and publications.)

Holistic Health Center
9201 Sunset Boulevard
Suite 501
Los Angeles, California 90069
c/o Pat Phillips, Coordinator of Services

(Offers comprehensive services encompassing medicine, psychology, art, movement, meditation, biofeedback, etc.)

The Women's Institute & Health Center, Inc.
7151 W. Manchester Avenue
Suite #1
Los Angeles, California 90045
c/o Dr. Marilynn Pratt
(Offers physical and psychological health care services. Focuses on a total health program for women, including basic education regarding the relationship of body to soul. Please include a stamped, self-addressed envelope.)

Body Independence Day
Independence Day Committee
Body Freedom Foundation
PO Box 2185
Minneapolis, Minnesota

The Holistic Life University
1627 10th Avenue
San Francisco, California 94122
(The Holistic Life University, which is approved by the State of California to conduct two-year certificate training programs, is part of the Holistic Life Foundation, a nonprofit educational organization dedicated to improving the quality and conditions of human birth, life, and death.)

Bibliography

BODY AWARENESS

Bartal, Lea, and Nira Ne'eman. *Movement, Awareness and Creativity.* New York: Harper and Row, 1975.

Brown, Barbara. *New Mind, New Body: Bio-Feedback.* New York: Bantam, 1974.

Feldenkrais, Moshe. *Awareness Through Movement: Health Exercises for Personal Growth.* New York: Harper and Row, 1972.

Fisher, Seymour. *Body Consciousness: You Are What You Feel.* Englewood Cliffs, N.J.: Prentice-Hall, 1973.

———. *Body Experience in Fantasy and Behavior.* New York: Appleton-Century-Crofts, 1970.

Gunther, Bernard. *Sense Relaxation: Below Your Mind.* New York: Macmillan, 1968.

Rose, Anthony L., and Andre Auw. *Growing Up Human.* New York: Harper and Row, 1974.

Rush, Ann Kent. *Getting Clear.* New York and Berkeley: Random House and Bookworks, 1973.

Schutz, William C. *Here Comes Everybody: Bodymind and Encounter Culture.* New York: Harper and Row, 1971.

Stevens, John O. *Awareness: Exploring, Experimenting, Experiencing.* New York: Bantam, 1971.

BODY CONTACT

Downing, George. *The Massage Book.* New York: Random House, 1972.

Hofer, Jack. *Total Massage.* New York: Grosset and Dunlap, 1976.

Inkeles, Gordon, and Murray Todris. *The Art of Sensual Massage.* San Francisco: Straight Arrow, 1972.

Leboyer, Frederick. *Birth Without Violence.* New York: Alfred A. Knopf, 1975.

———. *Loving Hands: The Traditional Indian Art of Baby Massage.* New York: Alfred A. Knopf, 1976.

Montagu, Ashley. *Touching: The Human Significance of the Skin.* New York: Columbia University Press, 1971.

Ribble, Margaret A. *The Rights of Infants: Early Psychological Needs and their Satisfaction.* New York: Columbia University Press, 1965.

Thie, John F., and Mary Marks. *Touch for Health.* Santa Monica, Calif.: Devorss, 1973.

Young, Constance. *Massage: The Touching Way to Sensual Health.* New York: Bantam, 1975.

BODY IMAGE AND ATTITUDE

Clark, Kenneth McKenzie. *The Nude: A Study in Ideal Form.* New York: Pantheon, 1956.

Fast, Julius. *Body Language.* New York: M. Evans, 1970.

Grenier, Cynthia. *The Nudity Thing.* New York: An Essandess Special Edition, 1967.

Guthrie, R. Dale. *Body Hot Spots.* New York: Van Nostrand-Reinhold, 1976.

Horn, Marilyn J. *The Second Skin: An Interdisciplinary Study of Clothing.* Boston: Houghton Mifflin, 1968.

Kern, Stephen. *Anatomy and Destiny: A Cultural History of the Human Body.* Indianapolis: Bobbs-Merrill, 1975.

Kleinke, Chris L. *First Impressions: The Psychology of Encountering Others.* Englewood Cliffs, N.J.: Prentice-Hall, Inc., 1975.

Kurtz, Ron, and Hector Prestera. *The Body Reveals: An Illustrated Guide to the Psychology of the Body.* New York: Harper and Row, 1976.

Lange, Ed. *Nudist Nudes.* Los Angeles: Elysium, 1964.

———, ed. *The Shameless Nude.* Los Angeles: Elysium, 1963.

Laver, James. *Modesty in Dress*. Boston: Houghton-Mifflin, 1969.

Lowen, Alexander. *The Language of the Body* (original title: *Physical Dynamics of Character Structure*). New York: Collier, 1974.

Nierenberg, Gerard I., and Henry H. Calero. *How to Read a Person Like a Book*. New York: Pocket Books, 1971.

Roach, Mary Ellen, and Joanne Bubolz Eicher (Eds.). *Dress, Adornment, and the Social Order*. New York: John Wiley, 1965.

Rudofsky, Bernard. *The Unfashionable Human Body*. Garden City, N.Y.: Doubleday, 1971.

Salkin, Jeri. *Body Ego Technique: An Educational and Therapeutic Approach to Body Image and Self Identity*. Springfield, Ill. Charles C Thomas, 1973.

Simon, Peter. *Decent Exposures*. Berkeley, Calif.: Wingbow Press, 1974.

Taylor, Gordon Rattray. *Sex in History*. London: Thames and Hudson, 1953.

Wilson, Robert Anton. *The Book of the Breast*. Chicago: Playboy Press, 1974.

BODY KNOWLEDGE

Belsky, Marvin S., and Leonard Gross. *Beyond the Medical Mystique: How to Choose and Use Your Doctor*. New York: Arbor House, 1975.

Boston Women's Health Book Collective. *Our Bodies, Ourselves: A Book by and for Women*. New York: Simon and Schuster, 1973.

Carlson, Rick J. *The End of Medicine*. New York: John Wiley, 1975.

Cassell, Eric J. *The Healer's Art: A New Approach to the Doctor-Patient Relationship*. Philadelphia: J. B. Lippincott, 1976.

Clendening, Logan. *The Human Body* 4th ed. New York: Alfred A. Knopf, 1974.

Gittelson, Bernard. *Biorhythm: A Personal Science.* New York: Arco, 1976.

Illich, Ivan. *Medical Nemesis: The Expropriation of Health.* New York: Pantheon, 1976.

Luce, Gay Gaer. *Body Time: Physiological Rhythms and Social Stress.* New York: Bantam, 1971.

McKenna, Marylou. *Body Power.* New York: Simon and Schuster, 1976.

McVerry, V. *The Family Self-Testing Health Guide.* Phoenix, Ariz.: O'Sullivan, Woodside, 1976.

Miller, Don E. *BodyMind: The Whole Person Health Book.* Englewood Cliffs, N.J.: Prentice-Hall, 1974.

Miller, Sigmund (Ed.). *Symptoms: The Complete Home Medical Encyclopedia.* New York: Thomas Crowell, 1976.

Palmer, Bruce. *Body Weather: How Natural and Man-Made Climates Affect You and Your Health.* Harrisburg, Pa.: Stackpole, 1976.

Sagov, Stanley E., and Archie Brodsky. *The Active Patient's Guide to Better Medical Care.* New York: David McKay, 1976.

Samuels, Mike, and Hal Z. Bennett. *Be Well.* New York and Berkeley: Random House and Bookworks, 1974.

———. *The Well-Body Book.* New York: Random House, 1973.

Sehnert, Keith W., and Howard Eisenberg. *How to Be Your Own Doctor (Sometimes).* New York: Grosset and Dunlap, 1975.

Stonehouse, Bernard. *The Way Your Body Works.* New York: Crown, 1974.

Vickery, Donald M., and James F. Fries. *Take Care of Yourself: A Consumer's Guide to Medical Care.* Reading, Mass.: Addison-Wesley, 1976.

BODY THERAPIES

Baker, Ellsworth. *Man in the Trap.* New York: Macmillan, 1967.

Barlow, Wilfred. *The Alexander Technique.* New York: Alfred A. Knopf, 1973.

Bean, Orson. *Me and the Orgone.* New York: St. Martin's Press, 1971.

Chesser, Eustace. *Salvation Through Sex: The Life and Work of Wilhelm Reich.* New York: William Morrow, 1972.

Feldenkrais, Moshe. *Body and Mature Behavior.* New York: International University Press, 1970.

Keleman, Stanley. *Your Body Speaks Its Mind: The Bioenergetic Way to Greater Emotional and Sexual Satisfaction.* New York: Simon and Schuster, 1975.

Kelley, Charles R. *Education in Feeling and Purpose.* Santa Monica, Calif.: Interscience Work Shop, 1970.

Lowen, Alexander. *Bioenergetics.* New York: Coward, McCann Geoghegan, 1975.

———. *Love and Orgasm.* New York: New American Library, 1967.

———. *The Betrayal of the Body.* New York: Macmillan, 1967.

Maisel, Edward (Ed.). *The Resurrection of the Body: The Writings of F. Matthias Alexander.* New York: University Books, 1969.

Reich, Wilhelm. *Character Analysis.* New York: Farrar, Straus and Giroux, 1972.

———. *Function of the Orgasm.* New York: Farrar, Straus and Giroux, 1961.

———. *The Sexual Revolution.* New York: Farrar, Straus and Giroux, 1963.

Rolf, Ida P. *Structural Integration: Gravity, an Unexplored Factor in a More Human Use of Human Beings.* New York: Ida P. Rolf, 1962.

Wyckoff, James. *Wilhelm Reich: Life Force Explorer.* Greenwich, Conn.: Fawcett, 1973.

NUDE BEACHES AND RESORTS

Elder, Leon. *Free Beaches: A Phenomenon of the California Coast.* Santa Barbara, Calif.: Capra Press, 1974.

Hartman, William E.; Marilyn Fithian; and Donald Johnson. *Nudist Society.* New York: Crown, 1970.

Ilfield, Fred, and Roger Lauer. *Social Nudism in America.* New Haven, Conn.: College and University Press, 1964.

International Naturist Guide. Ed. Fankhauser, and Rene E. Kielinger, eds. Naturisten-Verlag, CH-2075 Thielle, Switzerland, 1973.

Swenson, Jr., Rod (Ed.). *Nude Resorts and Beaches.* New York: Popular Library, 1975.

SEX EDUCATION FOR CHILDREN

Fleischhauer-Hardt, Helga. *Show Me: A Picture Book of Sex for Children and Parents.* Pictures and captions by Will McBride. New York: St. Martin's Press, 1975.

Mayle, Peter. *Where Did I Come From? The Facts of Life without Any Nonsense and with Illustrations.* Secaucus, N.J.: Lyle Stuart, 1973.

Nilsson, Lennart. *How Was I Born?* New York: Delacorte, 1975.

Salk, Lee. *Preparing for Parenthood.* New York: David McKay, 1974.

Sheffield, Margaret. *Where Do Babies Come From? (A book for Children and Their Parents).* New York: Alfred A. Knopf, 1975.

SEX EDUCATION FOR GROWNUPS

Colton, Helen. *Sex After the Sexual Revolution.* New York: Association Press, 1972.

Hatfield, Tom. *Sandstone Experience.* New York: New American Library, 1975.

Kass, David J., and Fred F. Stauss. *Sex Therapy at Home.* New York: Simon and Schuster, 1975.

Otto, Herbert A., and Roberta Otto. *Total Sex.* New York: Peter H. Wyden, 1972.

Index

Acupressure, 65
Aging, 8
Alcohol, use of, 27-28, 153
Alexander, F. M., 54-55
American Center for the
 Alexander Technique, 57
American Heart Association, 29
American Institute of Family
 Relations, 103
American Psychiatric
 Association, 60
American Psychological
 Association, 60
American Sunbathing
 Association, 153
Anatomy and Destiny,
 14, 16, 20
Association for Holistic
 Medicine, 41
Association for Humanistic
 Psychology, 41, 60

Babies, need for body contact,
 64-67
Baby Roll, 83
Baker, Ellsworth, 46
Bartholin gland, 18
Bathing, 111
Bathing, communal, 125,
 160-61, 193
Beachfront U.S.A., 151,
 199-201
Bean, Orson, 46
Beauty
 and cultural bias, 5-7
 and mass media, 7-8
Benedict, Ruth, 124
Berscheid, Ellen, 5
Bernstein-Tarrow, Norma, 98
Bindrim, Paul, 59-60, 62,
 63, 193

Bioenergetics, 48-50
Birth, Leboyer method, **66**
Black's Beach, 149
Blackwell, Elizabeth, 19
Body acceptance
 and self-esteem, 4-5, 11, 77
 teaching children, 90-93
Body Appearance Questionnaire,
 9-10
Body Attitude Questionnaire
 21-23
Body Calendar, 34-35
Body-Compliment Game,
 191-92
*Body Consciousness: You Are
 What You Feel*, 8
Body contact
 as basic need, 62-68
 children's need for, 64
 in primitive societies, 65
Body contracts, 102
Body Freedom Foundation, 207
Body games, 100
Body image
 correlation with self-esteem, 4
 negative, 1-9
 and relationships, 5, 6, 7
Body Independence, Declaration
 of, 205-12
Body-mind integration, 37-41,
 42-57
Body odors, 105-6
Body parties, 172-96
Body Reveals, The, 42
Body self-examination, 25, 32,
 111, 119, 139-40
Body taboos, 17-21
Body therapy, 42-57
Braguette, 126
Breast examination, 25
Breasts, appearance of, 129

INDEX

Breslow, Lester, 26
Brooks Beach, 149
Brothers, Joyce, 93
Browning, Elizabeth Barrett and Robert, 17

California School of Professional Psychology, 61
California State University (Long Beach), 60, 98
California Supreme Court, 198
Callen, Eugene, 199
Calvin, John, 15
Cardiovascular disease, 29
Center for the Healing Arts, 38, 39
Center for Marital and Sexual Studies, 103, 114
Childlike play, 82
Children
  evaluating attractive, 5-6
  and nudity, 90-102, 148
  and need for body contact, 64
Cigarette smoking, 27
Cinder, Cec, 151
Clitoris, removal of, 18
Club Mediterranée, 171
Codpiece, 126
Comfort, Alex, 133, 201
Conceal-Reveal Game, 178-80
Cromey, Robert, 203
Culture, and standards of beauty, 5-7

Dancing, 191
Dancing naked, 85-89
Deer Park, 60
DeLuise, Dom, 164-66
Dewey, John, 55
Dingwall, Paul, 36
Duncan, Isadora, 78

Eating properly, 28
Eating as a sensory experience, 84-85
Eden, 201-2

Elder, Leon, 146
Elysium Field, 70-73, 75, 157, 162-66, 201-2
Emotions and body prejudice, 16
Emissions, nocturnal, 19
Environment
  experiencing, 79, 83-84
  and health, 38
Erections, fear of, 127-29
Esalen, 59-60, 157, 159-61
Eupsychian Management, 60
Exercise, need for, 28-29

Facials, 190
Family relationships and nudity, 90-102
Fashion Show Game, 183-84
Feldenkrais, Moshe, 55
Feldenkrais Method, 55-57
Fisher, Seymour, 8
Fithian, Marilyn, 60, 114, 129
Fleishman, Stanley, 203
Floating Technique, 193-94
Four Seasons Nature Park, 154
Fraser, Kathleen, 1
Free Beaches, 147
Free to Love, 108
Freeman, Evelyn and Albert, 95-96
French Revolution, 16
Freud, Sigmund, 45, 92-93

Games, 191-93
Glen Eden, 151-52
Gordon, Sol, 94
Greening, Thomas, 37, 44, 158
Greenwald, Harold, 105
Group nudity, 122-24
Gunther, Bernard, 58

Harlow, Harry F. and Margaret K., 65
Hartman, William, 60, 103, 114, 129
Health, 11, 26-30

Holistic health, 36-41, 160-61
Holistic Health Center, 24, 40
Hot-tubbing, 193
Humanist, The, 78
Huxley, Laura Archera, 85

Ile du Levant, 155, 156
Indians and modesty, 125
Industrial Revolution, 16
Institute for Bioenergetic Analysis, 48
Institute for Family Research and Education, 94
Institute of Rehabilitation Medicine, 55

Japanese, The, 125
Japanese and modesty, 125
Journal of Humanistic Psychology, 37, 158
Joy of Sex, The, 201

Kelley, Charles, 50-51
Kern, Stephen, 14, 16, 20
Kurtz, Ron, 42

Lange, Ed, 70, 197, 201-2
Langley Porter Neuropsychiatric Institute, 36
Laver, James, 125-26
Laying-on-of-hands, 65
Leboyer, Frederick, 66
Lerner, Max, 172
Littrell, Richard, 103
Lowen, Alexander, 48-50
Luther, Martin, 15

Making Friends with the Opposite Sex, 74
Marks, Mary, 66
Maslow, Abraham, 60
Massage, 64, 80-82, 101, 185-87, 194-96
Masturbation, 18, 19-20
McClure, Sally, 83

Me and the Orgone, 46-47
Menstruation, 106
Modesty, 95-96, 124-26
Modesty in Dress, 125
Montagu, Ashley, 63, 66
"Move Like I Move" game, 192-93
Mueller, William, 80, 195
Mueller College of Massage, 80
Murphy, Michael, 159

National Center for the Exploration of Human Potential, 16
National Institute of Child Health and Human Development, 64
New Age Health Care Services, 36
Nude beaches, 148-51, 199-201
  foreign, 155
Nude cruises, 155
Nude Man's Buff, 192
Nude marathons, 60, 61-64
Nude resorts, 151-55
Nude travel tours, 155-57
Nudity
  and communal bathing, 125
  as educational tool, 73-74
  and erections, 127-29
  and family relationships, 90-102
  and fear of rape, 130
  and freedom from role-playing, 123-24
  group, 122-24
  guidelines, 96-102, 148
  and the law, 197-204
  learning to accept, 72-73
  and sexual intimacy, 103-20, 126
  social, 122-24, 172-96
  as therapy, 58-64
Nutrition, need for proper, 28

INDEX

Obesity, 25, 29, 130-32
Orgasms
 limiting of, 19
 superstitions about, 16, 18
Orgonomy, 46
Otto, Herbert, 16, 123

Paul, Jordan and Margaret, 96, 107
Penis size, 94, 105, 115, 129
Personality types, classifying, 48-49
Phillips, Patricia, 24, 40
Pierrakos, John C., 48
Pills, 31-32
Pirate's Cove, 149-50, 199, 200
Pratt, Marilynn, 34, 39
Preparing for Parenthood, 94
Prescott, James W., 64, 100
Prestera, Hector, 42
Price, Richard, 159
Primitive societies and body contact, 65
Psychology Today, 2

Radix education, 50-51
Radix Institute, 50
Red, White, and Blue Beach, 149
Reich, Wilhelm, 45, 205
Reichian therapy, 45-47
Rice, Ruth, 64
Rimmer, Robert, 78
Rockefeller Institute, 53
Rolf, Ida, 53

Rolf Institute, 53-54
Rolfing, 53-54
Rudofsky, Bernard, 122

Salk, Lee, 90, 94
San Gregorio Beach, 198
Sandstone, 157, 166-69
Sarty, Merrill E., 5
Self-acceptance, 11, 41, 123
 and nudity, 61-64, 114

in body liberation workshops, 135-46
and self-esteem, 77
Self-examination, 25, 32, 111, 119, 139-40
Self-massage, 80-82
Sense Relaxation: Below Your Mind, 58
Sensory feast, 84-85
Seward, Jack, 125
Sex, as "necessary evil," 18-19
Sexological examination, 114-20
Sleep requirements, 28
Sleeping nude, 107-8
Smith, Chad Merrill, 197
Social nudity, 172-96
 in Europe, 155
Song of Myself, 69, 135
Spock, Benjamin, 93
"Spermatorrhea," 19
Stone, Harold, 38
Stransky, Judith, 57
Strip Bean Bag game, 192
St. Paul, 14
Swenson, Rod, 151
Syphilis, 20
Syracuse University, 94

Teenage nudity, 96
Thie, John F., 65-66
"Tom Jones" dinner, 183
Touch for Health, 66
Touching: The Human Significance of the Skin, 63
Tranquilizers, 32

Unfashionable Human Body, The, 122
University of California (Los Angeles), 26, 44, 70
University of Southern California, 5
University of Wisconsin, 65
U.S. International University, 105

Vaginal secretions, 106
Victorian morality, 15-21, 125
Von Newman massage, 145, 185-89

Walling, William B., 48
Walster, Elaine, 5

Wheatley, Paul, 61-62
Whitman, Walt, 69, 135, 204
Women's Institute and Health Center, 34, 39

You Are Not the Target, 85